TOUCHING
HORSES

TOUCHING HORSES

COMMUNICATION, HEALTH AND HEALING THROUGH SHIATSU (Acupressure)

Marion Kaselle and Pamela Hannay

PHOTOGRAPHS AND ILLUSTRATIONS BY MARION KASELLE

Appendix on holistic veterinary medicine
with Allen M. Schoen, DVM, MS

J.A.ALLEN
London

British Library Cataloguing in Publication Data
A catalogue record for this book is available from the
British Library

ISBN 0.85131.579.8

Published in Great Britain in 1995 by
J.A. Allen & Co. Ltd.
1 Lower Grosvenor Place
London SW1W 0EL

Typeset in Hong Kong by Setrite Typesetters Ltd.

Printed in Spain by Printeksa SA

Contents

*For the Horses
and their Caretakers*

Acknowledgements

Marion Kaselle

I thank Max, Katydid, Red, Stardust, and Judy Mann for their love, support, patience and honest editing.

I thank Katydid, my task-master, for her lessons in quantum mechanical physics and metaphysics.

I thank her and Pamela for teaching me about energy and healing, and for asking me to write this book.

I thank Dr Allen Schoen for his generous attention and contributions, and Dr Meredith Snader for her assistance with the meridian diagrams.

I thank New York Film Works, my photo lab, for giving service the old-fashioned way, which is sadly too rare today.

And I thank Loretta Van der Veer and Beth Sproule for allowing and helping their beautiful horses to pose for the photo-diagrams.

Pamela Hannay

To Florence Warner, for the first push toward a horse who needed me, and for their confidence.

To Wataru Ohashi, for his words, 'Don't press, just be there.'

To Marion Kaselle, for gently taking me by the hand and strongly pulling me toward this goal.

And to Richard Aschoff, whose love makes everything better.

AUTHORS' NOTE

This book is not intended to replace proper veterinary diagnosis and treatment and should not be used for that purpose.

The authors are not responsible for any personal injury that may arise while performing these techniques. It is assumed that the reader is fully aware of the dangers and risks inherent in working with and around horses. It is assumed as well that the reader takes full responsibility for such risks, for learning and practicing common-sense safety precautions, and for understanding that, in spite of such precautions, the unpredictable can and does still happen in an instant.

HORSE CREDITS

The black Dutch Warmblood stallion **Sauvage Diamant** appears in the following diagrams: muscles of the shoulder, skeletal system of the hindquarters, LI-Lu meridians, B-K meridians, and the TH-HC meridians. He was United States Dressage Federation Horse of the Year – Training Level in 1989 with 74%, and has been Grand Champion of numerous prominent breed shows. He is also the sire of Katydid's beautiful foal, Shadow King, born in May 1993. He is owned by Loretta Van der Veer of River Foal in New York.

Perseus modelled the acupressure points for the forearm, the shoulder, the hindquarters, and the feet. He is an Oldenburg-cross, bred, owned, trained and ridden by Elizabeth Sproule. He was 1988 Zone II Insilco Horse of the Year – Training Level, 1989 Eastern States 1st Level Champion, 1990 Zone II Insilco Reserve Horse of the Year – 2nd Level, and 1991 Quebec Medium (4th) Level Champion. In 1992 he was showing successfully at FEI levels.

Kir Royale appears at three months old in the diagram for the spinal column and back muscles. He is a Dutch Warmblood by Sauvage Diamant out of Diva, owned by Loretta Van der Veer and Sheree Hall.

Foreword 1

by Marion Kaselle

It was spring, the ground was once more forgiving and green, and my mare and I were exercised to fitness. I loaded her into my brand new trailer, attached to my brand new tow vehicle, to follow my trainer to our first show of the season. However, our book didn't read as the script in my dreams. The brand new trailer was defective, and so began a far different journey than I could have planned.

The ill-designed trailer, without warning, flew into a violent snaking track. It threw my mare back and forth across a highway, first upright, then on its side and hers. It won the pull and took me with it. In the aftermath, our real injuries were invisible, and comparable.

Finding help for my human ills proved far easier, if less forgiving, than for those of my mare, Katydid. I turned to the alternative health care resources to which I long had been committed: my doctor, who is a homeopath and nutritionist, a chiropractor, a masseur, and a shiatsu practitioner. I was readily diagnosed and treated for whiplash and trauma, though it took the additional help of a Gestalt therapist before my body would respond.

The traditional care attending Katydid could find no cause for her symptoms. She was therefore diagnosed to have a behavioral or attitude problem, in spite of it being newly acquired and completely atypical, and in spite of a diminishing physical capacity that told me otherwise. The veterinarians shrugged; the trainers shrugged and called for spurs; I looked elsewhere for help; Kate grew worse. As she sought to preserve her rhythm and balance, her problems compounded: from first losing fluid movement and roundness over fences, to switching leads, cantering stiffly inverted, jerking her neck, and seeming unwilling to work, to losing virtually all forward movement but bending her neck to the left until her lip rested on my boot's toe. Four months following the trauma, while I still searched for alternative care, an 'inexplicable' splint developed, and did not want to heal.

Six months down our uncharted journey, Kate's splint seemed re-covered. But a half-hour's exercise brought subtle lameness. The sports massage techniques, that I applied from a book, did help topically, relieving certain symptoms, but they obviously weren't reaching the source. Stiffness now claimed her long fluid walk; pain and frustration claimed her spirit.

We then met Pamela Hannay. After our brief greeting, she placed a hand over Kate's "third eye" and said, "Hello, Katy. Do you have a headache?"

She had immediately seen the source of my mare's woes – a neck vertebra forced severely out of alignment by the trailer's wild gyrations. The bone stuck out, I could see, now that I understood what I saw. The barn manager/trainer with a degree from Cornell had not seen it, nor four veterinarians – this is understandable: our eyes had not been trained to see this way. The displaced bone had by now caused a misalignment of her back, the recurring subtle lameness, and all other symptoms she had suffered – all compensations for a displaced neck.

Pamela began to work. Within minutes she realigned Kate's back and restored her fluid walk. She worked for two hours, taking breaks that allowed Kate to feel the changes in her body and make further adjustments on her own. When the session was over, that severely displaced vertebra was back where it belonged, and Kate and I both knew that she, at last, was on the path to being well.

Pamela gave us more than a physical treatment and emotional relief: she showed me her basic shiatsu techniques so I could continue to guide Katydid through healing. Twenty minutes of her time put an invaluable ability literally in my hands. My hands became tools to simply, gently, effectively promote healing in another being; they became tools of communication, to listen and to speak, to sense and move energy, to stretch and move muscles and limbs and awaken them to unknown possibilities. Pamela brought us light.

At first three times per week, then twice, then when needed, I applied shiatsu techniques to my mare. Initially tentative, but knowing that through these I couldn't hurt her, my hands and eyes and instincts grew in confidence and competence. When the neck vertebra again slipped out, I was able to detect it and help it back to alignment; when Kate deposited my saddle from her back into the aisle, I understood pain had returned and how to proceed. Her frustrations diminished as my comprehension grew.

Although I had always spent extensive time with Katydid, beyond training and care, the quality of our time now deepened. I had observed her, but now possessed the means to understand what I saw. I had pursued a rapport, but did so now through a rich and tactile vocabulary, and through a new realm of awareness that is shiatsu. My human arrogance slipped away to allow me to see what had always been: that my mare was my teacher. My confidence in working with her continues to grow, as I continue to "listen". And, so importantly after the trauma we shared, I regained confidence in my own instincts.

Katydid is the kind of horse who is always "getting into trouble". Always alert, inquisitive, independent, reactive and testing, she is an equine Sarah Bernhardt. She is also what, in the terms of this book, I would call 'a *Yang* type with much *Yin*': actively outgoing, yet extremely sensitive and temperamental. She affords me, almost daily, the opportunity to entwine the philosophy and techniques of shiatsu into her care and training, and into our relationship. Together, slowly, we learned and still learn how to adapt techniques and ourselves to each other.

Calmly I tell her she's rude and obnoxious, as I stroke her neck and kiss her cheek. She continues to be. I lead her out of her stall and allow her to lead me in zig-zags until she'll stop at the cross-ties without a fight. This only takes a minute. Now it's down to China she digs, until I still her with a firm hand and voice: my touch says, "I understand, but that's not acceptable." She gives me her leg, but glares with flattened ears. I teasingly chide, push forward her ears, and continue to groom. My grooming the other horse first has, as usual, provoked her. I don't want to fight with Kate. Her aggressions brush by me, through air, and tumble softly to ground. Before I've finished, she is once again my agreeable angel, affectionate and responsive. We are both at peace.

What I give Kate through shiatsu comes back a thousand-fold. There are times when I don't feel well that Kate needs shiatsu treatment – by the session's end I invariably find that I feel measurably better, somewhat healed. Often I detect and treat the early signs of a problem. I know joy each time I see the relief in Kate's body from the work of my hands: her softened eyes then seem to know of miracles. I have learned to "be" in the moment, which is the entry to experiencing joy, and other wonders. I know the thrill of my mare moving before or beneath me in the fullness of her beauty and grace, a vibrant athlete once more. Beyond health we have gained a deep sense of well-being and confidence, a knowledge and ability to self-heal, and boundless access to each other and the universe.

Without Pamela's work, or that of someone like her, Katydid would have been lost to a permanent shadowy lameness. Until the source of her problems, the displaced vertebra, could be detected and corrected, a compounding need for bodily compensations would persist to deteriorate her health and spirit. My beautiful, talented, beloved mare would have been discarded and destroyed, and needlessly. Before our detoured journey, I met too many horses with this fate. And I wonder, sadly, how many could have been saved by the right eyes and hands.

This book is an offering, out of my experience and daily practice of shiatsu with two horses, a pony and a friend, and out of the knowledge of Pamela, who is a true healer. It is an offering to her species from Katydid, who was implored to forgo the green grass at her feet to pose for our photographs, and whose suffering and trust carried us along our journey to this light. We hope that the information in this book will benefit and enrich your horses, your lives and your relationships, as it has our own.

Foreword 2

by Pamela Hannay

Animals have always been a source of fascination, knowledge and joy for me. They are purely sensitive beings with whom we share our purest emotions. They are my teachers. So when, in 1983, someone asked me to help a severely injured horse, it was a welcomed gift. It at once seemed the answer to my prayers for a new direction in my work, one that would wed the art of healing with the love and affinity I had always felt for horses.

The injured horse, Lexington, a six-year-old thoroughbred, had displaced his neck and back by falling over backwards eight months before our meeting. His pain and disablement had progressed to the state where he could not be groomed, he could not graze, and he acted with aggressive hostility. Yet he seemed to accept me. I knelt in a corner of his stall. I made myself small, non-threatening and humble. I wished to be used as a channel for healing and for a sign that it was permissible to begin. I was soon aware of warm breath on my hair and velvet lips on my cheek. Our healing time had begun. I allowed my hands to intuitively move to various points on his body and, while doing this, was aware of him moving to so present me with areas where, I understood, he needed help. After half an hour of touching and gentle movement of his head and neck, he was able to graze for the first time in eight months. The joy and amazement I felt at this moment was indescribable. I think he, from that moment on, associated me with the absence of what must have seemed endless and oppressive pain. The next day, after more movement, pressing and bending of his neck, his head tilt was gone, and I saw the headache leave his eyes. We held each other's gaze for a moment of infinity. We thereafter worked twice a week. In three weeks his body returned to balance, his attitude improved. In six weeks he was able to be ridden for the first time since his injury, moving beautifully, correctly. He soon resumed jumping.

So Lexington was my first teacher for this new aspect of my work. He patiently guided me to the way to rotate and stretch his legs, to stretch his back by pulling his tail, to the way to translate my knowledge of healing the human "bodyminspirit" to that of the equine.

My impressions begin when an owner calls asking for help. In my mind's eye, I often see where the problem is before I'm told, by seeing a specific area of the horse's body. Learning to trust my instincts hasn't always been easy, but it is always the correct way to work. When I first meet a horse, I can sense where he hurts, what he does to compensate, and sometimes even know when it happened. When we meet I quiet myself and become his for that time. I mentally tell him that whatever he wishes to share will be respected. I extend myself to him as pure love. The responses are always interesting and moving. Often I'm flooded by a certain emotion, or by images of events that perhaps proceeded an injury or caused it. I believe this type of information is available to all of us; however, some have learned, through desire and patience, to become better "listeners".

I work with many attitude problems. This also means working with the people who created them. Sometimes we work on very old patterns. Always we work in an atmosphere of trust, respect, understanding and support.

Some of the most beautiful moments happen in workshops where people bring their horses to learn how to work with them in this way. They find old injuries they weren't aware of, sometimes correcting them almost at once. Mostly, they gain a new perspective, a new awareness of their horses' bodies and beingness, a new way to communicate with them. They develop a sensitivity that often has far-reaching positive benefits in other areas of their lives. Their horses may ask for attention to an area where they were never comfortable being handled. The horses too learn new awareness of their bodies, a fuller mobility and a sense of wholeness, well-being, and ability to self-heal.

Animals know our intentions and will rarely refuse help from us, unless a memory is too painful. We must show them the respect they deserve, allow them to fulfil their potential, and open ourselves to their gifts. Each horse I have worked with lives in my heart and continues to be my guide.

Introduction
The Benefits of Shiatsu for Your Horse . . . and You

Horsemanship is an art and a privilege, as most of you reading this know and appreciate. It is the essence of communication, and of beauty, as well as a means to transcend and transform ourselves. The consent and cooperation of a horse allows us this experience. My horse guides my pursuit of this art, while shiatsu has become my most valued tool. Shiatsu serves the art of horsemanship and fulfils the responsibility that privilege holds.

Shiatsu is a gentle, deeply effective, holistic system of health care. It comes to us from Asia, out of a system of thought and practice that has been developing for over 5000 years. It is an empirically proven, deeply knowledgeable, highly sensitive, and yet simple system. It is non-invasive and safe to administer. It is used to restore health, and to maintain it. It is a way to "see". It is rooted in the philosophies and theologies of the East that see the universe as a dance of energy manifesting itself into the life forms, matter and forces that we know: all is energy, all is interconnected, and each unit is inextricable and vital. Modern physics and medical research now concur with this view.

Pamela Hannay studied the system of shiatsu with Japanese masters. Since 1978 she has applied its techniques successfully to treat humans. In 1983 she was given the opportunity to translate and develop these techniques to benefit the horse, an effort that has become the prime focus of her work. She has proven to many Westerners what the Chinese long have known, that the highly sensitive being we call "horse" is at least as, if not more, responsive to this healing art as are humans. Pamela and a handful of practitioners consistently demonstrate the inestimable value of this healing system, as they bring our horses back to a state of health.

Many of the horses Pamela treats come to this healing form as a last resort, having failed to respond to our Western systems of diagnosis and cures. Some are suffering severely, others marginally but enough to detract from their tractability and performance.

Modern Western medicine and thought are rooted in the doctrine of rationalism, in the philosophy of Descartes, and in the discovery of the microscope, all of which sprang forth in the mid-seventeenth century. Rationalism regards "reason", rather than experience or "sense", as the source of absolute knowledge. Descartes, a proponent of rationalism, used "reason" to separate, with absoluteness, the mind/soul from the body, and to affirm that animals are soulless: the human body and the entire animal were reduced to models of machines. The microscope facilitated this view, by drawing our eyes and understanding to the pieces of life, in increasing minutiae, as our sight and "sense" of the whole receded with the decades.

Our Western mechanistic world view, born of the scientific and philosophical leaps of the seventeenth century, was overthrown in this century by quantum mechanical physics ($E = mc^2$, electromagnetism, light waves, radio waves). Yet it has bequeathed us a medical system based in the overthrown theories: that living beings are as machines with fixable parts, and that matter, rather than energy, is the "real" and prime component of the universe.

With the exception of homeopathy and naturopathy, Western medicine developed to treat disease, and more often merely the symptoms of disease, rather than focusing on the patient as a unified, indivisible whole governed by an energetic life force. The tools of this matter-based system are drug therapy and surgery. Although we are increasingly adept at breaking down matter into its molecular components, so to better target these therapies with less destruction to the entire organism, orthodox medicine often falls short of achieving optimal health. When diagnosis and treatment succeed, we often must then recover from the "cure", from the "side-effects" of drugs, and are left with an internal struggle to regain equilibrium.

Orthodox medicine treats symptoms that define a disease in order to treat the disease. Without diagnosis, treatment is stymied. The subtle first signs of ill-health often do not provide enough clues for treatment until they develop into a blatant problem. Even then, the signs must fit into some known category before treatment can commence. You or your animal must be suffering, and from an identified illness, before you can receive help. All humans and animals have symptoms that do not fit into a recognizably treatable illness, i.e. one described in medical and veterinary texts. So most of us have, at some time, been frustrated by a doctor's or a veterinarian's failure to diagnose a problem or restore full health. And most of us have experienced drug therapy side-effects, sometimes as discomforting and debilitating as the symptoms or disease cured.

Drugs are designed to lessen or eliminate symptoms, not to eliminate the disease that caused them and that will continue to cause symptoms to appear. Some drugs are designed to wipe out an invading offending organism, but this necessitates damaging more than that organism in the process: "... if penicillin is to be a medicine for human beings, it must have the power to alter the health of human beings, and not only of bacteria."* Unlike missiles, we cannot direct drugs to attack only their target.

All drugs alter the patient's inherent healthful processes, including the immune system. These alterations are termed the "side-effects" of drugs. One profound side-effect is that drugs silence symptoms that are messages from the body and mind and are part of the healing matrix.

* Richard Moskowitz, MD, *Homeopathic Reasoning* (San Francisco, 1980), p. 5.

A "running" nose is the body's removal of an offending virus and the inflammation it has caused. A sensation of pain is a call for help; it's a survival mechanism, as is the release of endorphins, the body's own pain-killer. So maintaining your pained horse on a drug such as phenyl-butazone, or giving your crying baby a sedative, may give your eyes and ears silence, but your horse or your child, and you, retain the problem – it's a "quick fix" that doesn't fix, but serves to sustain ill-health.

Holistic medicine seeks to restore and maintain the health of the patient, rather than attack the disease. It views the patient as an intricate network of subtle energy, and diagnoses the subtle to gross imbalances within. The practitioner stimulates and guides this energy to re-establish the equilibrium and harmony that is health. Shiatsu administers no drugs, creates no negative side-effects. Problems that are not diagnosed, even ones that do not yet show visible symptoms, and problems that do not show up on x-rays nor in medical textbooks, can be treated. The first subtle signs of disease can be attended to, before they develop into disease.

> "It is easy to dissolve a thing when it is yet minute.
> Deal with a thing while it is still nothing;
> Keep a thing in order before disorder sets in."
>
> *Lao Tzu, Tao Te Ching,* Chapter LXIV, lines 152–152A, translated by D.C. Lau,
> Penguin Books Ltd (London, 1963), p. 125.

Regular treatments of shiatsu bestow multifold benefits. Regular stimulation of the healing potential maintains a well-tuned immune system. Accidental injuries, even severe ones, will heal more quickly. Muscles, joints and connective tissue are made and kept supple, reducing physical stress, reducing susceptibility to injury, and maximizing physical potential. The stressed or nervous mind learns to relax with the body, and nervous habits, including pre-performance jitters (horse and human), diminish. The dull and listless patient becomes energized. The patient learns to communicate with his/her own body with an increasing awareness of the potential within. And with this awareness, the self-confidence of the patient grows.

With improved health, the shiatsu patient becomes more sensitive to imbalances within, in the same way that you become aware of a speck of dust, not noticeable on a dirty surface, but apparent on a clean one. This is true for both humans and horses. We become increasingly sensitized to our needs and to our ability to maintain our health. My mare now asks for (sometimes demands) my help, with a sore muscle, an undetected injury, or an indigestion. She has a heightened awareness of her body, its boundaries, its potential, and the sensation of well-being. She has learned how to activate her own healing potential, with my assistance or through her manipulations. I've seen her in the paddock repeating the leg rotations and stretches that I've performed with her, and I've seen her pull the tips of the pony's ears when he was ill as she watched me do. I've watched her when I knew she didn't feel quite right, as she seemed to listen intently to her body and make the necessary adjustments.

Shiatsu can benefit the healthy, the half-healthy and the ill. It is useful for the new-born, the professional, the pet and the retiree. Touch is vital to the mare-foal relationship, to the new-born's sense of security and place. Shiatsu's touch can attend to the foal's health and ease him/her into the human world, instilling trust and love and tractability. A yearling, raised from birth with shiatsu, recognized something in my greeting touch and immediately pressed specific points of her body – apparently sore from a day of intense play – into my hand. The physical and mental stress common to performance horses can be reduced to manageable proportions, minimizing injuries and maximizing potential with greater consistency. Through the shiatsu techniques of stretch and rotation, and the elimination of stiffness, soreness and pain, horses are able to expand their physical limits. The relaxation and revitalization effects of shiatsu can be used according to need before and following performance. The pet and the retired horse can be relieved of old injuries, of stiffness and soreness, of arthritic pain; they can be given renewed or new flexibility, new or renewed ways to move and feel.

Shiatsu is performed by the sensitive use of the hands and an ever-growing awareness of the dynamics affecting the patient. The intentions, the sensory and intuitive knowledge of the practitioner, as well as the depth of learned technique, factor the practitioner's capacity to influence the healing potential within another. But the basic techniques are easily learned and performed, and even an initiate at a first attempt can produce a visibly positive response, if not a dynamic one.

Familiarity with shiatsu techniques will expand your language of touch. It is a means of profound communication, one to which horses are especially responsive. From birth, horses associate touch with a sense of security and communion. Their sense of touch is highly evolved and extremely sensitive, even to the emotions and intentions of others. The loving and healthful nature of the shiatsu techniques are welcomed by horses. Even a moment of shiatsu treatment, as you're entering or exiting a class, asking for a new training maneuver, or attempting to pass the monster spotted pig on the trail, is a relaxed, pleasurable moment of sharing and nurturing trust. Horses learn and heal faster, and perform better, without the presence of fear or pain.

Shiatsu can treat common but evasive problems that often bewilder owners, trainers and traditional veterinary care, such as shortened or incorrect movement, stiffness, elusive lameness, temperamental sensitivities, and problematic temperaments and behavior. An "inverted" stiff neck carriage, resistance to flexion, a loss in balance, a lack of roundness, stumbling, travelling on the forehand, switching leads, reluctance to work, resistance, a dull and listless attitude, an argument-ative temperament, maniacal behavior, nervousness, headshyness, earshyness, tailshyness, biting, bucking, rearing, being "off" – all are among familiar complaints that persist after rider, training and con-formation faults have been ruled out, and after your very competent

INTRODUCTION ———————————————————————————————— *xxi*

veterinarian and farrier have scratched their heads and tried their full battery of tests and treatments. Most of these "enigmatic" symptoms are due to undetected injury and pain, including the mental pain of environment stress.

With shiatsu treatment, physical and many behavioral problems can disappear with the pain. You most likely will discover, or recover, a happy and willing companion in your horse, and a depth of gratitude in her eyes. In the process, you, the practitioner, will become more aware of your own energy, your behavior and other influences upon your horse. You will be able to deal with problematic attitudes and behavior caused by environmental stress and lack of human understanding. Nervous habits such as cribbing and weaving may be reduced, possibly eliminated if the stress and cause can be removed, and if the habit can be broken. New understanding and habits may supplant the equine instinct of flight. Trust and knowledge may supplant fright. Shiatsu techniques may replace artificial training devices. A cooperative partnership can revoke the politics of power. With halter and lead line in your hand, soft, warm breath may replace the mud and heels in your face. Your horse will be safer and more pleasurable to work with. Your veterinarian and farrier will thank you.

Shiatsu does not replace your veterinarian. It cannot replace your veterinarian's specialized knowledge, experience and skills, but should be an eminent partner in healing and health maintenance. Shiatsu may identify and alleviate problems before they escalate and suggest traditional medical intervention. In emergencies it offers non-invasive first-aid techniques while you await the doctor, so to lessen shock, decrease heat, increase circulation, and alleviate stress, without the use of drugs that will disguise symptoms and hinder diagnosis and healing. Shiatsu can speed recovery from critical ailments, such as lameness, some colics, and "tying-up" syndrome, sometimes profoundly, again without drugs. For an injured leg, passive exercise is applied with the body relaxed and the leg supported by the practitioner, so muscles are exercised without the stress of weight-bearing, circulation is increased, and healing is accelerated. Shiatsu, applied regularly, will also discourage the formation of painful scar tissue. Even with the use of drugs and surgery, shiatsu can greatly enhance the healing process. And, as already said, shiatsu can eliminate shadowy lamenesses and ailments that elude orthodox medicine. The balance you create between shiatsu, related holistic therapies*, and traditional veterinary care will be uniquely deter-mined by your horse's current state, history and nature, and the realities of your life.

Relaxation, of both the patient and the practitioner, is a primary effect of shiatsu treatment, crucial to healing. A relaxed body and mind lets go of its limitations and opens itself for healing, for communion with another being and with its own healing power. Shiatsu (and acupuncture) effects the release of endorphins which block the sensation of pain, so the body and mind can transcend pain to a relaxed, elevated state and healing can occur. Relaxation allows energy to flow freely through the

* There are now veterinarians professionally trained in the related holistic therapies of acupuncture, chiropractic, homeopathy and herbal remedies. An explanation of these modalities and sources for certified veterinary practitioners are given in Appendix B.

body and mind. A shiatsu session is revitalizing, leaving the patient and the practitioner both relaxed and energized. Relaxation and health are infectious. When other horses watch a treatment being given, they relax and respond.

You, the practitioner, will benefit as much as your horse. You'll know the gratification of effecting your horse's health. You'll discover the healer within and yourself as an invaluable resource. You will learn to trust and use your instinctual knowledge. Your ability to observe and understand will expand and deepen. Your self-confidence will grow. A heightened sense of security, and intimacy, will inform and enrich your daily care. You'll be able to respond more and more to your horse's needs, thereby fulfilling your own. You will further cultivate some qualities of the good rider: awareness, being centered, being "there" (concentration), and the ability to sensitively "listen" and communicate through feel.

The practice of shiatsu will inform and enrich your relationships: with your horse, with yourself, with all life forms, and with life itself. The communication that crosses the boundaries of species and the boundaries of skin, that exists between man and animal, human and horse, man and man, has a very powerful beauty, a beauty that heals, a beauty that is joy.

How to Use this Book

Our book offers a system of techniques that will help your horses heal and stay healthy. The system has been proved through 5000 years of practice and further confirmed by current medical and scientific research. The techniques are *safe*, *simple*, *easy* and *quick* to learn and perform, requiring merely the use of your hands in a gentle, natural way. There's nothing complicated or difficult about shiatsu. The simplest, most natural techniques, not deep painful pressure, work the best. A treatment can take as little time as five to ten minutes, or up to ninety minutes to administer to a compounded condition.

This is not esoteric knowledge. Oriental medicine does have such levels, but they are not pre-requisites of healing. You can, in fact, use these techniques to help your horse without understanding their principles. But an explanation of those principles and the system they govern is given here for interest. The concepts of Oriental medicine have been simplified so as not to confuse or overwhelm the beginner. Readers seeking deeper understanding will find numerous suitable texts. Our primary purpose is to introduce this system of healing techniques for horses, as transposed by Pamela Hannay from those for humans, to horse owners and handlers, for whom many of these concepts will be new. Veterinarians, acupressure therapists and owners of other pets will also find our book useful. Our aim is to offer you enough information so you can give the most benefit. The information is here for you to take from as you need and wish.

The book is organized into three sections:

□ SECTION I: **Some Definitions**

This section explains the common terms of shiatsu and the underlying principles of this system of health.

□ SECTION II: **Techniques**

○ "Moving Energy" explains the touching and stretching techniques.

○ "Evaluating Problems", "Feeling Energy", "Quieting a Nervous Horse" and "Touching Pain" will help guide you to do just what these chapter titles say.

○ "Keeping Your Horse Whole" gives ways to enhance your treatment sessions.

○ "Treating Kyo and Jitsu" explains more advanced theory and treatment, but may help the beginner to evaluate and treat some conditions.

○ "The Environment" and "Preparing Yourself" suggest ways and means of enhancing treatment and of you personally giving and getting the most from it.

☐ SECTION III: **Shiatsu Treatment**

This final section gives details of shiatsu treatment of the entire horse, of specific areas, and for specific problems.

We know that many people have limitations of time, and that your horse may have a problem wanting immediate attention. If this is so, turn to the chapter in Section III that focuses on the problem area, or to the "Index of Specific Problems", or, if you don't know what specifically is wrong, to "A Shiatsu Massage: Diagnosis and Treatment" and to "Evaluating Problems". You should read "Feeling Energy", "Moving Energy", "Keeping Your Horse Whole", and any other technique chapters that you feel specifically apply to your situation (possibly "Touching Pain"). You should also read, in Section III, "Treatment Guidelines" and "A Shiatsu Massage: Diagnosis and Treatment". Looking up unfamiliar terms in Section I will facilitate your understanding.

Of course, we hope that you will read all of *Touching Horses*, and that its parts add up to a greater whole.

An understanding of shiatsu and holistic medical thought offers alternatives and a vital means to restore and preserve health. This does not mean that we discard the knowledge and advances of Western traditional medicine – we *expand* on them. By taking responsibility for our own health and that of the animals in our care, we gain a deeper understanding of health, disease, and the differing choices possible for every individual. We assume your commonsense ability to know when to call your veterinarian for his/her areas of expertise and treatments, and how to integrate shiatsu into the full picture of your horse's care. *You* decide the balance and nature of that integration, based on the realities of your life, your horse's individual nature and state of health, and the knowledge available to you – from all the bright sources you can find!

Dr Allen M. Schoen is an internationally prominent veterinarian now limiting his practice and teaching to the alternative therapies of acupuncture, chiropractic, homeopathy, herbs and nutrition. In Appendix B: Holistic Medicine in Veterinary Practice, he defines these therapies and his holistic approach. Addresses are provided of the professional societies through which to locate veterinarians certified in the respective therapies. Dr Schoen works with conventional veterinarians and through referrals by them. He stresses the importance of a *balanced* approach to health care and maintenance: "We must use our best judgments while remembering that the animal's welfare is our main concern. Whatever modality works best for that animal in that situation is the one that should be used. The key to being a good healer is to know the indications and the limitations of what you do, to know when one modality is appropriate and when one isn't. All of the therapies, alternative and conventional, have their place and *work together* for the *animal's* best interest. Shiatsu is not a replacement for the benefits of veterinary care, both conventional and holistic. It is not a cure-all, a panacea, a rainbow. It is one of the tools we can use in the healing of animals and ourselves."

SECTION I

SOME DEFINITIONS

1 *Shiatsu*

In Japanese, **shi** means "finger" and **atsu** means "pressure". Literally **shiatsu** means "finger pressure", a pressure that gently stimulates the body's natural healing ability.

For longer than recorded time, touching techniques have been employed by social animals to relieve pain and to promote and maintain health and vitality. The very physical interplay that occurs naturally among horses, beyond serving as social dialogue, attends to their health. Using their sensitive and strong lips, horses, like other animals, engage in mutual massage and grooming sessions. It becomes clear while watching such a session that each horse is able to make her own needs known and fulfilled by another as she presents various body areas for stimulation.

Medical research has disclosed that our skin is the largest producer of hormones and immune cells in the body. This is a partial explanation of the profound healing effects touch can produce. A hug, a touch or the stroke of a hand will stimulate the production of vitalizing hormones and immune cells.*

For over 5000 years, the Chinese have depended on a system of healing and preventative medicine known to us as acupuncture. It employs stimulation to specific receptive points on the body so to rebalance the vital energy field within. *Anma*, which in Chinese literally means "press-rub", was the first point-pressure therapy, using touch as the precursor to needle insertion. Acupuncture in time developed to produce a more profound effect, but a continuous tradition of "acupressure", or "acupuncture-without-needles" was established as a companion therapy. All forms of acupressure and massage are based on the principles of Chinese medicine (even "Swedish massage", so-called because a Swede introduced it to the West!).

The underlying principle of the Chinese medical system is the field of subtle energy, **Ki**[†], that governs the cellular level of living bodies through an intricate system of channels called **meridians**. The smooth, continuous, balanced flow of Ki through the meridians provides optimal health.

Acupressure is not the "laying-on-of-hands", which refers to the healing power of intensified subtle magnetic energy produced in the hands of people sometimes called "psychic healers". And, unlike some other forms of touch therapy, acupressure is not directed at the nervous system or the muscular system, though it influences these as a secondary effect of the Ki energy in the meridians. The production of hormone and immune cells in the skin is, likewise, a secondary effect of the activation of Ki, part of its healing-force matrix.

* Deepak Chopra, MD, *Quantum Healing Workshop*, 1990.

† The Chinese know it as "Chi" or "Qi".

3

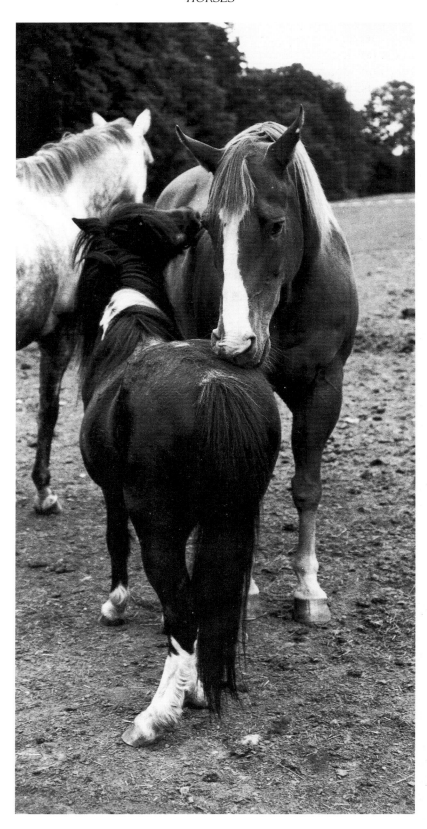

Red is applying deep, circular pressure with his upper lip along the pony's croup. Stardust, the pony, is doing the same for Red at his mid-section. This ritual is regularly performed after dinner, as they present each other with varying body areas. Kate, in the background, awaits her turn. She often appears for breakfast with her neck and back muscles covered in grassy mouth stains.

Shiatsu is a form of acupressure from Japan, to which country the Chinese medical knowledge was imported. Shiatsu, simply, is a system of medicine that restores and maintains the health of the patient by moving and rebalancing the vital Ki energy within with the touch of one's hands, with "finger pressure".

Energy

The past century has seen the emergence in Western thought and science of a new way of "seeing" our world, a way that leads on a direct path to the philosophy and science of the East. The orthodox Western system for 300 years, that of the rationalism of Descartes and Newton and their model of the universe as a "Great Machine", could no longer correctly answer questions posed by scientists delving into the phenomena of electromagnetism and light and heat, the world of subatomic particles. Quantum mechanical physics emerged with the answers and, to the dismay of even their discoverers, astoundingly toppled the foundations of Western rational thought.

Our commonsense and our senses have been dethroned as the dictators of "reality". Our physical world has been exposed as essentially one of illusion. Quantum physicists dived into the world of energy and discovered that energy is the world.

Energy, in constant motion, constructs the universe. It is what we are made of. Matter, the physical world perceived by our senses, is not the solid "reality" most of us believe in. Matter is composed of atoms, atoms of particles, and particles are now known to be "energy packets" (quanta), never at rest, constantly fluctuating. All particles are in a unified field of energy, which is the universe. Energy is all there is, in continuous motion and transformation.

Particles of energy form electromagnetic (EM) waves. The EM waves are differentiated by frequency. We experience them as light, sound, heat, and radio waves. A color is a frequency of light. As our senses perceive only a very limited area of the frequency range, the "real" look of the world lies beyond our physical boundaries. And as the human sensory range differs from those of our fellow animals, another creature's sense of "reality" will be very different from ours, and just as valid – or invalid. Our world of matter is of low-energy frequencies, slow enough to seem solid and stationary. Our bodies are actually integrated electromagnetic fields, vibrating at low frequencies, and integral (and convertible) parts of one unified field.

Ki Energy and Meridians

Ki energy is subtle energy. Subtle energy has higher frequency than matter. It is beyond our normal perceptual range and, until recently, that of our scientific instruments.* Ki is perceived, in research results as well as in Oriental medicine, as the essential life force. From conception, it governs the development and ordering of the cells into the physical

* An increasing number of researchers believe that subtle energy moves faster than light, placing it in a domain of negative space/time and making it primarily magnetic and generative (retains order without decay) in character. This being so, it transducts down to lower-frequency EM waves (but higher frequency than matter) in our physical bodies. It is then these secondary EM waves that our new refined instruments are recording. Energy moving faster than light is a well-regarded and "proved" theory that remains beyond our technical capability. (Richard Gerber, MD, *Vibrational Medicine*, Sante Fe, NM, Bear & Co., 1988, pp. 143–153.)

forms of life we know. It continues as the governing life force through an intricate system of channels known as **meridians**. Through the meridians, every cell in the body is directed by the subtle Ki energy. It is a negatively entropic force, which means that it maintains order, as opposed to decay — it is a force to preserve the "blueprinted" life form. When Ki leaves the physical body, death occurs and the body decays (is now entropic).

The continuous and balanced flow of Ki through the meridians is essential to optimal health. A disruption in this flow is the source of dis-ease and eventually disease. When the flow of Ki is interrupted, through blockages in the meridians for example, the physical body stops functioning properly, and gradually breaks down if a balanced flow is not restored. New instruments (able to detect higher-frequncy EM fields) have confirmed that a disturbance in the energy in the meridians *precedes and predicts disease.* They further show that acupressure or acupuncture applied to the meridians restores a balanced flow and health. The diagnostic readings taken with these instruments are the equivalent of those taken by the shiatsu or acupuncture therapist through the sense of touch.

Research headed by Professor Kim Bong Han, and duplicated by Pierre de Vernejoul and many others, has confirmed the existence, primacy, function and the location of the meridians as reported in Oriental medicine. It has also confirmed the location and receptivity/conducivity of the cavities in the skin known as the acupuncture points (*tsubos* in the Japanese language of shiatsu). The meridian system was found to form shortly after conception and before the development and formation of the organs. It was found closely linked with the cell nuclei of the tissues, the endocrine and the nervous systems. The stimulation of an acupuncture point causing the release of endorphins (our natural pain-killer) is demonstrative of these relationships. Fluid extracted from meridian channels contained uniquely high concentrations of DNA, RNA, amino acids, and many hormonal substances such as adrenalin and corticosteroids. A common error assumes that the nervous system and the meridian system are one and the same, and that Ki is the nerve pulse — but research has visually confirmed the meridian system as separate and unique, as well as sovereign over the molecular and cellular systems of the living body.*

The meridians comprise an interconnecting network of superificial and deep channels that run throughout the body. The superficial pathways lie one-eighth of an inch to four inches beneath the surface of the skin. Above them, occurring at intervals, are the acupuncture points (tsubos).

There are fourteen major pathways in the body. They are superficial with deep branches reaching to the major organs and connecting directly with each other. It is the superficial branches that treatment is applied to, and that are drawn on our charts of the meridians.

Two of these major pathways are called "vessels".† They run midline and meet at both ends to form a continuous loop around the body. In the horse, the **Governing Vessel** (GV) begins in the hollow under

* Gerber, pp. 122–127, 185–198. Gerber summarizes this research and gives original source references within his text.

† There are actually eight vessels, all considered reservoirs of Ki, but traditional treatment emphasizes the two we mention.

the base of the tail, runs under the tail bone to its tip, then traces the dorsal (upper) midline to the upper gum of the mouth, where it meets the termination of the **Conception Vessel** (CV) tracing the ventral midline from below the anus. They are considered the most important reservoir of Ki in the body, and the regulator of the flow of Ki through the twelve organ meridians. The Governing Vessel carries nourishing Ki to the spinal cord and the brain, governs the **Yang** organ meridians (which will be explained shortly), and can increase the Yang energy of the body. The Conception Vessel nourishes the uterus and genital system, governs the **Yin** organ meridians, plus the Stomach Meridian (a Yang channel), and can increase the body's Yin energy.

The twelve other primary meridians are organ-related and linked with one of the twelve main bodily functions. They are bilateral, each being actually a mirror-image pair — a branch on one side of the body has an identical twin tracing the same path on the other side. Ten of these meridians are named after the body's ten major organs, and so are the **Lung** (Lu), **Large Intestine** (LI), **Stomach** (St), **Spleen** (Sp), **Heart** (H), **Small Intestine** (SI), **Bladder** (B), **Kidney** (K), **Gall Bladder** (GB) and **Liver** (Lv) meridians. The names refer to the realm of *function* that they govern, not to the structural organ. The remaining two major meridians are named after two bodily functions that are defined in Chinese medicine, and are called the **Heart Constrictor** (HC) and the **Triple Heater** (TH).*

Each of the organ-related meridians begins or ends on a finger or toe in humans — six to each hand and foot. In four-legged animals this translates to six meridians beginning or ending on each front and hind foot. Half of each group runs along the outer (lateral) surfaces of the legs and half along the inner (medial) surfaces. The six meridians on the outer side (three on the front legs and three on the hind) all run between the head and the feet; they are classified as Yang. The six meridians of the inner legs run between the feet and the interior of the body: they are classified as Yin. The twelve meridians are paired, a Yin with a Yang, an inner with an outer, according to their complementary functions. Yin and Yang are explained more fully in the next chapter and in Appendix A: Notes on the Twelve Major Meridians.

YinYang

In the nature of Ki energy, as in everything, is the duality known as **YinYang**. Yin and Yang are names for the two polar aspects of one thing, such as night/day, female/male, in/out, and the negative and positive poles of a magnet. They coexist in an interplay of balance which is constantly revolving. Through cyclical movement, one and then the other will predominate, will appear and pass as the sun and moon in our skies. When you pass through the entry of your home, the influence of its exterior and interior are momentarily in balance, as night and day at dawn and dusk; once inside, the interior environment envelops you, though the exterior surface simultaneously exists and

* Due to the difficulties of translating Chinese concepts into Western thought, these two meridians are known by a number of interchangeable names: the **Heart Constrictor** is also called the Pericardium (P), Circulation Sex (CX), Heart Envelope (HE), and Circulation (Cir); the **Triple Heater** is also called the Triple Burners (TB), Three Warmers (TW), and San Jiao (SJ).

exerts some spatial and material influence; the one cannot exist without the other, though at most moments it is one or the other that most affects you. So it is with Yin and Yang.

Yin is characterized as the inner, quiet, receptive female principle. Yang incorporates the male principle of expansion, creation, restless activity striving toward fulfilment. They are relative qualities, not absolute.

Oriental medicine defines each of the organ meridians by its YinYang nature, and couples them accordingly. The coupled organ meridians are complementary in function and mutually supportive. Their YinYang designations further describe the nature of each and their relationship. The Yin organ meridians seek to sustain homeostasis, to store, not drain; the Yang meridians generally function to drain rather than store, to transform nutrients and dispose of waste. The bladder, a Yang organ function, is coupled with the kidneys, a Yin organ function: both are involved with bodily fluids and purification, but one deals with more external, superficial-level functions and the other with more internal, deep-level ones. Imbalance/disease in one of the paired meridians will usually affect the other. The Symptoms Index of Meridian Correspondences in Appendix A charts the qualities, relationships and prime functions of the twelve organ meridians.

Awareness of the YinYang designation of a meridian aids the practitioner in interpreting subtleties in the balance of the Ki energy within. There is always some Yin quality present in the energy with Yang, and some Yang with Yin, and, as explained, the balance is in constant flux. Yet, disturbances in that dynamic balance occur, in the intensity or quantity of Yin or Yang, in the rhythm and timing of their ebb and flow, and it is these subtle qualities in the energy that the experienced shiatsu practitioner seeks to detect and reorder.

Balance Equals Health

When the Ki energy flows rhythmically, harmoniously and unimpeded through the meridians, it is found to be in balance and the individual in health. A balanced energy flow is both the cause and the effect of good health. Blocked energy first creates imbalance, then illness. It is first experienced as a subtly reduced ease of motion, a stiffness, a slight ache, a vague throb at the temple or twinge in the stomach, a sense of worry or distress. It becomes increasing degrees of pain, physical discomfort, mental stress, that grows into disease and disability. Many factors can impede energy: structural misalignment, over-stressed muscles, dietary imbalance or irritation, stressful personal relationships, environmental stress (lack of turn-out, an unventilated stall, irritating noise). Shiatsu practice restores flow and balance to the Ki energy. The body's natural healing processes are activated, and balance is restored to the physical and emotional body of the individual. This balance is known as optimal health.

"Bodymindspirit"

Ki energy sustains and integrates our physical, mental and spiritual aspects, and so Oriental medicine deals with the body, the mind and the spirit of an individual, not as separate parts, but as an indivisible and unique entity, as a unique **bodymindspirit**. Our emotions affect the functioning of our organs, our organs of our limbs, our limbs and organs our emotions and our sense of well-being, physical pains and discomforts change our moods and our sense of ourselves, and our skin speaks of much of this. Horses, being of the same substance, prove this maxim as well. We often judge the health and well-being of a horse by the condition of his coat. *The Book of Lieh-Tzu*, an ancient classical Chinese medical text, expresses the sense of this:

> "My body is in accord with my mind, my mind with my energies, my energies with my spirit, my spirit with Nothing. Whenever the minutest existing thing or the faintest sound affects me, whether it is far away beyond the eight borderlands, or close at hand between my eyebrows and eyelashes, I am bound to know it. However, I do not know whether I perceived it with the seven holes in my head and my four limbs, or knew it through my heart and belly and internal organs ..."*

The shiatsu practitioner looks at and honors the horse as a whole individual and considers her habits, her temperament, her diet, her environment, her owner, her fitness level, her physical activities, any deviations within these, and all symptoms. No judgements are made, no blames assigned, no segmentations defined; there is no "bad leg" or "off leg", only what the bodymind of the horse says of the imbalance within and its attempt toward health.

Kyo and Jitsu

Two conditions characterize unbalanced energy within the pathways: voids and blockages. The voids are called **kyo** and are points or areas lacking and in need of energy. Blockages are areas that have drawn too much energy. They interrupt the flow and distort the balance. They are over-concentrations of energy, and are known as **jitsu**. An inflammation is an example of a jitsu condition.

Most often, the kyo is the first cause that produces the jitsu. The jitsu then becomes the physical manifestation of the problem, to be known as a "symptom". It is the Ki energy's attempt to compensate for a need it cannot fulfil.

One example of kyo producing jitsu is hunger. If your horse is always fed in her stall at 7 a.m. and one day hay, grain and water don't arrive until noon, she has stood in need for five hours. Her body is wanting nutrients, fiber and water, and her mind is wanting certainty that they will arrive. The physical and emotional stress created by the need of the

* Translated by A.C. Graham, PhD; John Murray Publishers Ltd, (London, 1960) p. 7. This ancient Oriental view, of the indivisible connection of everything in the universe, is in full accord with the maxims of quantum mechanical physics and the unified field theory.

digestive system will cause energy to rush to the areas responding to stress, which will be determined by the predisposition of the horse. Energy, in its efforts to restore equilibrium, will pool in these areas, that are now jitsu. Muscle spasms and colic may develop.

It is said that a kyo condition always underlies jitsu. Restoring Ki energy to points and areas that are void or depleted, that are kyo, is crucial to healing.

Kyo is treated with "tonification", the technique that sends warmth deep within the body to nurture strength and normalization. Jitsu is treated by stimulating points and/or areas with "sedation" techniques.

Source Versus Symptoms

The bodymind of the horse wants to be in health, in balance, in harmony within itself and with its environment. "Symptoms" are the physical manifestation of this inner struggle of the energy.

But symptoms are not the source of a problem. Removing the symptom(s) will not remove the problem, and new symptoms will arise as expressions of new energy dams and detoured flows, for the void is still void of the needed energy and the balanced flow is not yet restored.

Shitatsu does not treat symptoms, but seeks the removal of their source. Practice promotes an awareness of health and balance that may eliminate symptoms by eliminating their cause, long before symptoms become apparent and then disability and disease.

In the absence of awareness of the horse's normal behavior, temperament and physical condition, of her bodymindspirit, one can easily overlook the signs of stress until symptoms are screaming. You may notice that she is not as lively as the day before, that today she doesn't "want" to do a shoulder-in to the left, and that she bucked and jerked her neck on the right lead — "just didn't want to listen!" And you blame it on her temperament, or on her hormones, and shrug it off. When she's slightly "off", you notice, you rest her, but you cannot find the problem. The "off" becomes a lameness. You call your veterinarian, who takes x-rays with a thorough examination, gives bute, a ten-day rest order, and no findings. Ten days later she's still lame, now depressed, and so are you.

In the stress of a training session or a slip in the paddock mud at full gallop, a muscle is overcontracted or overstretched, and the fibers tighten into a tiny knot. This slight weakening and limitation of movement is not noticeable at first, but continued use aggravates and enlarges the spasm, causing pressure which brings discomfort and pain. The cumulative aggravation will bring a time when the muscle can no longer accommodate its task, even within its normal safe range of motion, and it will tear, or go into crippling massive spasm, or allow the breakdown of an associated tendon or joint. The original knot is the cause that must be undone, but at this point the ripped tissue is screaming for help and will receive the now needed treatment. When it heals, a problem will remain, and the horse will return to severe injury if the cause is not dealt with. (A regime of bute is not dealing with it.) The imperative of looking beyond symptoms to their source becomes clear.

"Protective splinting" is a form of the cumulative aggravation described above. It is the body's attempt to protect an injured area and regain balance through compensation, but the process also serves to spread the stress and damage while delaying total breakdown. An injury in a lower leg would cause an overload on the muscles of the upper leg, which, when their stress became too great, would be aided by the muscles of the shoulder or the hindquarters. You now have a very stiff and lame horse, whose problem *appears* to be in the shoulder, hip or hock. Symptoms and problems can also travel in the other direction, down from the neck, shoulder or back, creating eventually severe injury in a lower leg and leaving a hidden trail to its origin.

The shiatsu practitioner seeks to eliminate the source of ill-health. Through observation and through touch, she/he "listens" to the energy of the horse, then moves the energy to remove blockages and fill voids. The immediate goal is to reinstate flow so the unimpeded Ki energy can perform the healing process. You may not know the source of your horse's problem, but the energy within her does. The horse is much more than the sum of her parts.

Tsubos

Tsubos are the acupuncture points. They are minute to small receptive areas – 1–2 mm in diameter – upon the skin, with physiologically lower resistance to energy (greater electrical conductivity) than the surrounding skin.* According to classical theory, there are five "gate" points with the highest conductivity: in humans they are at the top of the head, the centers of the palms, and the bottoms of the feet; in horses, we surmise that they are between the ears at the crown and on the soles of the hooves by the apex of the frog.

The tsubos are aligned over the superficial branches of the meridians, and allow ready access to the Ki energetic system. Subtle energy as well as therapeutic stimulation may enter through these portals. Finger pressure, hair-width needles, electrical currents, sound waves, and low-energy laser beams used at specified points effect therapeutic changes within the meridian system and the physical/mental body. The gentle pressure of shiatsu, while not as physically profound as its sister therapies, can be deeply effective because it activates energy. The energy is the messenger within the body.

In Pamela Hannay's practice of shiatsu, as is illustrated in this book, therapy is focused on the meridian lines, rather than on the points, to activate Ki and re-establish a continuous, balanced energetic flow. You therefore do not have to concern yourself with the precise location of the tsubos, except for a number that prove very useful (for colic for one, shoulder tightness for another, and so on). Specific point-therapy is used with discretion. As you become sensitive to areas of kyo and jitsu, your touch will naturally be drawn to the tsubos.

* With new high-frequency sensitive instruments, various researchers recorded nearly twenty times less electrical resistance at the tsubos. They found the electrical conductivity to vary with the physiological and emotional changes of the human subjects. The tsubo points only appeared in electrographic scans when disease was present or proved imminent in their associated organs. Changes in the brightness of the points was found to "precede the changes of physical illness in the body by hours, days, and even weeks". The recorded radiant size and brightness of the points correlated with the acuteness of the disease. (Gerber, pp. 127, 178, 188.)

2 *Touch*

Touch is shiatsu's tool. Through sensitive nerve endings in our fingers we are able, through practice, to feel energy in ourselves and in others. All life – humans, animals, bugs, birds, fish, plants, even amoebas – pulsates with Ki energy. This force creates us, sustains us and unites us. We are of the same substance and, in essence, are one.

When you place your hands upon your horse, your energy and hers join and converse. Horses are very aware of this. It is a way they sense and know us. It is how they know we are nervous or tense, assured and calm, callous or warmly sensitive, and much more. This ability of horses is innate. So it is within humans, but with the emphasis on rationalism in Western education, most of us soon lose the ability, until we consciously seek to retrieve it. We can learn to know another through our sense of touch.

There are varying qualities and quantities to touch. A touch may be energetic but sensitive and soft, or soft, limp and dull; it may be full of angry energy, or protective – callous and withdrawn or defensively forceful; or it may be confidently forceful. Some touch is full of love and respect, another wants for both. A slap or a thump is the attempt of some people to connect with another on any level. There is also the slap to awaken awareness, as the Zen master to his pupil. A horse may throw you to send you into consciousness, or for more selfish reasons. Our touch tells much about us as individuals. And by developing the sensitivity and knowledge of it, we may learn many things about others.

How important touch is to our sense of well-being, how important it is to make physical/energy contact with other beings. We hug, hold and stroke each other. We hug, hold and stroke our pets, to fill an emptiness, to enhance a moment, to find a momentary calm center within the turbulence about us.

When our skin nears that of another, our energies mingle, are perhaps excited and warmed or repelled and chilled. Our like natures meet and converse. We unite with life outside of ourselves, a momentary dispelling of our illusion of aloneness.

To embrace another being is to embrace the very fabric of life, to feel the same force that creates and sustains us all, and all that we know (and don't know) in the universe. It is a reconfirmation of ourselves.

So we hug, shake hands, touch shoulders, slap, punch, kiss, go touch dancing, and, ride horses. We ride horses to join with this magnificent other creature. Through our seats and thighs and legs and hands, through the horse's back and sides and mouth, we carry on energy conversations that travel through our entire bodies when we allow them. Momentarily we may know the power, grace and gift of flight that is Horse. More

importantly, we may reach outside of ourselves to become one with
another.

Through the practice of shiatsu, we reach outside ourselves to feel
and affect the energy of another, to facilitate the natural healing process
within that other for the restoration and maintenance of his/her health,
to converse with and know him/her deeper than words, deeper than
skin, deep to the fiber that weaves us all to the fabric called Universe.

3   *Intuition*

Intuition is expanded awareness.

The information we seek moves before and around and inside us, in
the unified field. It has been said for millennia by seers and poets of the
East and West, it is now said by physicists and medical researchers:
every particle in the universe, every molecule in our bodies, every one
of us has instantaneous access to all of the information in the universe.
All we need do is drop the conceptual boundaries we ourselves have
constructed, our self-defined limitations. It is a fact that most of us
receive less than one-billionth of the stimuli available to us at any one
moment – because of *learned* perceptual commitments.

As with our knowing touch, intuition is an innate ability that most
of us are taught early to mistrust and lose ready access to. It is not
intellectual. It operates outside the walls and cause-and-effect rules of
reason and experience. The dictionary calls it instinctive knowledge or
insight. Insight means inner sight. It comes from within us, or through
us, from consciousness in the unified field of energy. It is a category of
knowledge that "just comes to you", as a sudden knowingness. It comes
to all of us.

Intuition sees, hears, knows beyond the limits of our senses and the
calculations of our minds. It is an endless resource – its limits illusionary
and self-created. It is deeper than our doubt, but doubt deadens its
voice.

The question, then, is how to hear your intuitive knowledge and
know it when it speaks. The answer is to first quiet yourself enough to
"hear". Open yourself without expectations, without judgements, without
"trying". Welcome it. Allow it to come. And when it does, acknowledge
it, trust it, trust its wisdom, "listen".

4 *Horse*

"For the animal shall not be measured by man. In a world older and more complete than ours, they move finished and complete, gifted with extensions of the senses we have lost or never attained, living by voices we shall never hear."

(Henry Beston, *Outermost House*, Garden City, Doubleday, 1929)

When we look at Horse, do we see him?

When Man sees Horse, he sees a being quite other than himself, but an other who has shared and shaped the course of human history for over 6000 years and into this century, a species that has surrendered his body to serve Man in partnership and in dreams, and yet remains obscure. In the face of the purported power of our intellect and superior brain capacity, and in spite of an inseparable relationship for thousands of years, Horse stands largely outside of our comprehension.

When most of us look, at anything or anyone, we see a reflection of our own thoughts, preconditions, wants and fears. We see through the mirror of our self-image, through the voices of our learning and the forces of our culture, through a curtain of illusions that we accept as reality.

Our axial illusion is that Man is the center of the universe. We've become an egocentric race, a race with an arrogant, narrow, obstructed vision, a vision that ensures our ignorance. From this position, we judge and rule over what we believe is "our" world. It's a position based in fear, a fear based in insecurity and incomprehension. The fear is of whoever and whatever does not reflect our individual version of the world. It is a fear of "Otherness".

Nature is the prime "Other" of Man, the feared power yet to be contained, unpredictable and untamable, answerable to its own Master who is not Man. We are in constant battle to control Nature, in our environment and within ourselves. We are taught to fear our natural impulses, our "animal nature", and to devalue our instincts.

Horse, more than any other animal, is Man's metaphor for Nature: stubbornly autonomous, often only a line away from wildness, respondent to a set of laws outside the bounds of human reasoning. Horse stands as a potent force of Nature to be bridled, controlled, dominated, much like the forces and calls to freedom within ourselves.

Horse, *Equus Caballus*, is the manifestation of over twenty-two million years of evolution (Man first appeared, by estimate, a recent 100,000 years ago). When the ancestor of our modern horse found his habitat evolving from woodlands and jungles with soft ground and leafy plants

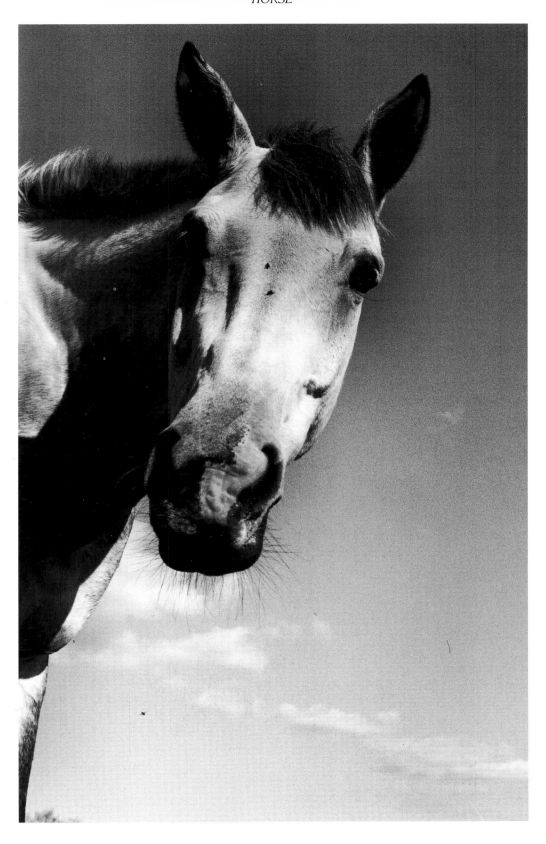

When we look at Horse, do we see him?

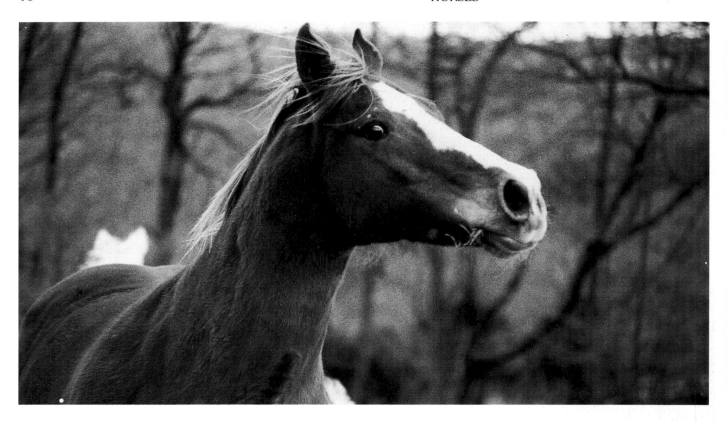

*Horses' acutely developed
senses of hearing and smell
bring them information
unavailable to us.*

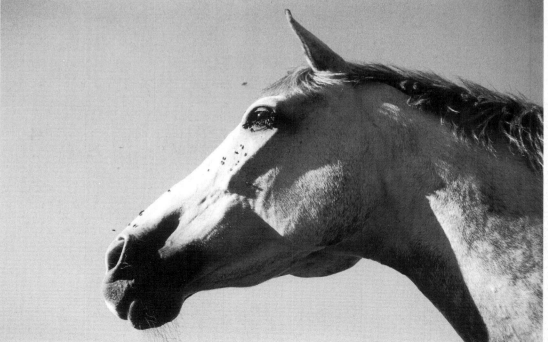

to open plains with tough, wiry grasses, he evolved corresponding adaptions that insured his species' survival. Horse became a grazing animal, equipped to process small amounts of roughage-type food gradually and continuously. He formed into a cohesive herd society with strata, roles and rules. Against enemies he evolved acute sensory apparatus to warn him of danger, and the instinct and speed for flight. These adaptions remain integral to his character. But they are incongruent to our convenience, and they are a repudiation of our domination and ingenuity. Our breeding programs may alter his physique to suit our eyes and needs, but we cannot divert his essence, that which makes him Horse.

Horse evolved senses he could believe in, and he evolved because he did and does believe his senses. This characteristic causes confrontation

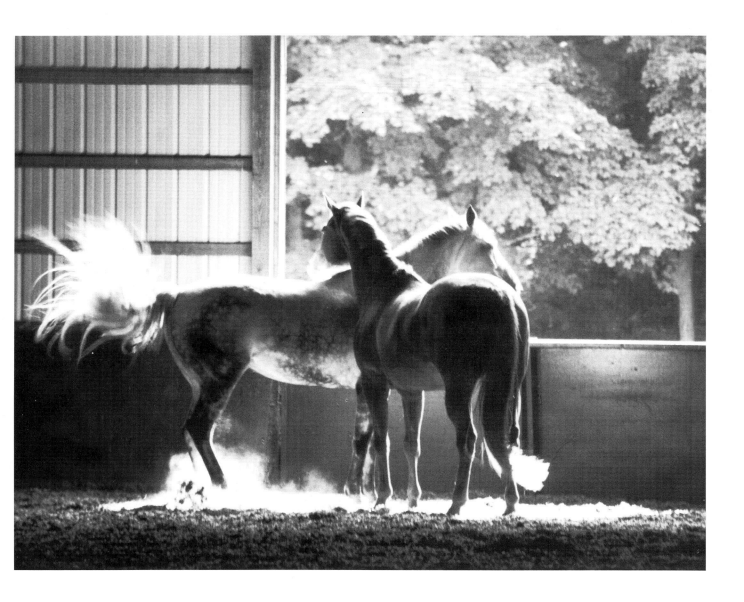

with Man, who presently values the rational powers of the mind and distrusts his own far-less-developed senses. We often find a human confused, frustrated and irate from her horse's response to an apparent nothingness.

Horses have their own culture and their own form of language, of which humans remain largely ignorant. They have access to knowledge which we mostly don't need, and which they now mostly don't need, but that is integral to them and to "... a world older and more complete than ours ...." When we dissolve the barriers of our vision, we see horses demonstrate high intelligence, sensitivity and deep emotional capacity, all of which is congruent with their own culture and not measurable by our own.

If you open yourself to the expressive body language of horses, you may see that the average horse finds the average human to be "dumb" and "irrational" (their versions of what we call "dumb" and what we call "irrational"). In language that seems perfectly clear to a horse, they silently "speak" to our uncomprehending sensory systems.

We take Horse out of nature, out of the environment he evolved to live within, and put him in our human world, as an object of our human visions and needs. We segregate him into individual stalls and paddocks, to protect our investment. We feed him a daily hay ration of a few flakes of alfalfa or whatever, because we've heard that it's "the best", which leaves him to spend most of his day standing within barred and solid walls with nothing to do, and his twenty-two million-years-old digestive

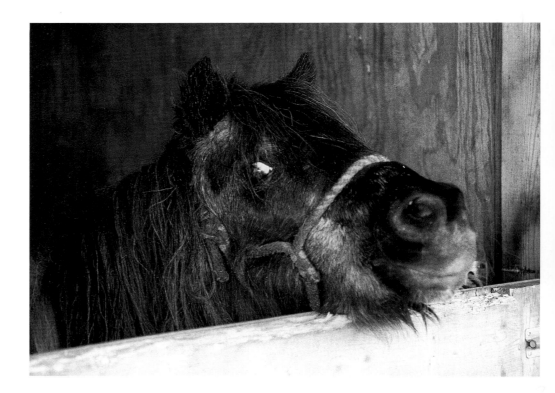

system in want. We wrap him in sheets and insulated blankets to save us time in grooming and cooling, to preserve the color and sheen of his hide, and to assure ourselves that we are caring. We insist on medicating a scrape, against his protest, to satisfy "our" need to "do something", ignoring the body's ability to self-heal. We wrap his legs to preserve their strength, ignoring that the legs of Wild Horse are never wrapped, legs that evolved to thunder over hard and rough terrain.

Beyond proper nourishment and shelter, and beyond health care to counter their disturbed ecology, horses have the need to survive with their nature intact, to live within the harmony of their cell memory, to live with a sanity only they can define. Our unwritten contract with the horse we have domesticated and bred demands that we nurture his sanity. Nurturing the sanity of horses demands that we both acknowledge and embrace them as Others; it demands that we open our visions to see Horse, rather than a dim, romantic or mechanical projection from the realm of human illusions. In the process, we will nurture our own sanity, we will nurture ourselves. Vicki Hearne, in her book *Adam's Task* (New York: Random House, 1986), so rightfully states that "... to be fully human is to recognize everyone and everything in the universe as both Other and Beloved ...." (p. 264).

If we want to share in the fullness of Horse, we must be aware that, to the degree that we impose our restrictive fears and constricted visions upon his management, handling and training, we increase his stress and diminish his spirit. To the degree that we deny his "horsehood", he is vulnerable to stress-related injuries, illness and behavior. To the degree that we do not honor his senses, his needs, his instincts, and his individuality, we deny who and what he is, and risk reducing him to a dull, mechanical mount, a resistant mount, or an insane, ummountable renegade.

Horses work for us when they work with us, through mutual understanding and mutual respect. A partnership is formed, not out of fear, but out of an earned mutual "right to command". Vicki Hearne addresses this right in *Adam's Task*:

> "What gives us the right to say 'Fetch!'? Something very like reverence, humility and obedience, of course. We can follow, understand, only things and people we can command, and we can command only whom and what we can follow." (p. 76)

If we encase our animals in false but convenient labels, such as "difficult", "dumb", "fractious", or "hopeless", we forfeit knowing the fullness of their beauty, the brightness of their souls, and the expansion of their potential into vibrant reality. To tame another requires allowing oneself to be tamed, which requires acknowledgement of the Other and a participation in open dialogue. It requires an investment of time and effort, rather than an expenditure of time and stress to perpetuate personal and cultural myths and preserve walled-off eyes and ears.

People and animals tend to fill out our visions and fulfil our prophecies, for better and for worse. We subconsciously shape the behavior, the performance, the mental set of whomever we exert our "power" over, including our children and our animals. We thus influence those in our custodial care and our relationships with them. So often we shape them with our fears and needs. We can, rather, acknowledge and nurture each as a separate, distinct, and wondrous individual.

> "He [the famous Alsatian dog Strongheart] forced me to realize that the making and breaking instrument in all my contacts with him was my own thinking, my own state of mind, my own inner attitude. Not his thinking or his state of mind or his inner attitude – but mine. I saw that I was primarily responsible for whatever happened in our relationship, and that the responsibility lay not so much in what I said or did but in what I really was up to 'mentally'."
>
> (J. Allen Boone, *Kinship With All Life*, New York, Harper & Row, 1954, p. 81–2.)

To summon our horses to the fullness of their beauty, which is also the fullness of their potential, we must first earn "the right to say 'Fetch'". A failure to do so is the failure to "see" and embrace the horse as Horse. By opening ourselves, our "visions", we attain "awareness" and self-knowledge, which are the basis for all true knowledge; we dispel ignorance, fear and our own isolation; we touch others and Others and begin to know the riches of our universe. Horses have so much to say to those who "listen".

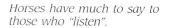

Horses have much to say to those who "listen".

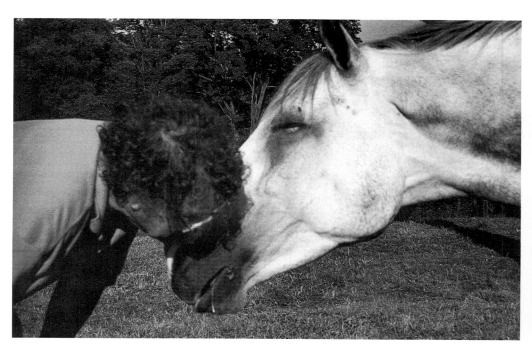

SECTION II

TECHNIQUES

*A horse's roomy, ventilated
and well-lit stall, where she
feels safe and relaxed,
makes a good working
environment for shiatsu.*

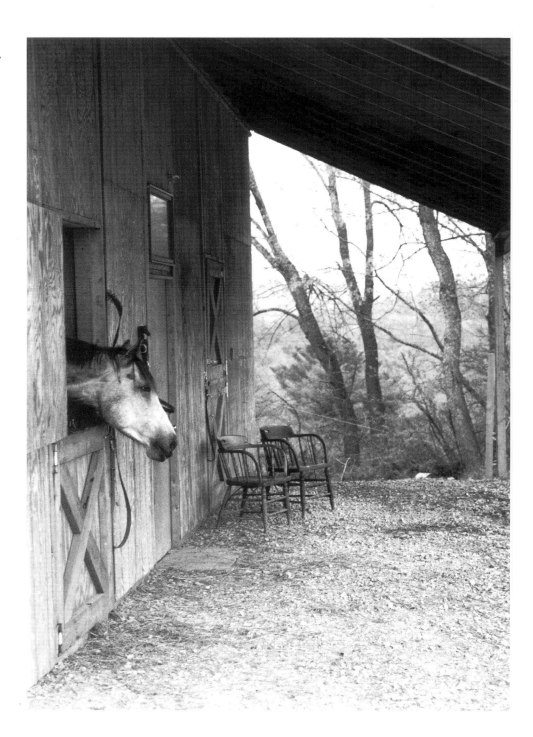

5 *The Environment*

The Physical Environment

Find a place to work where both you and your horse will feel comfortable, safe and at ease. Horses generally feel safe and relaxed in their own stalls, which makes them a good place to work if they are reasonably roomy, ventilated and well lit. If a stall is unsuitable or unavailable, work in a quiet corner of the barn, arena, yard, field or turn-out shed.

Because you want your horse to be able to move her body in response to your work, it is best if she can be unrestrained or on a lead line, rather than on cross-ties.

Try to work in a peaceful environment. You will want to find a quiet area, as free as possible from noise, traffic and distractions. Music and chatty friends may relax you, but consider your horse. It's doubtful that loud or jarring music or conversation will soothe her nervous system, and it will most likely distract you both. Let the other people in the area know that you will be working with your horse, and request that they respect your needs for a limited time. If possible, you might avoid working during the normally busy and noisy times around the barn, the times of frequent shouts and clattering pails, bangs and thuds, hurried foot-falls, and expected feed. These precautions, beyond enhancing a healing environment, can help you avoid injury from a startled horse.

Be aware of your horse's state of mind when choosing your work area and time. Consider the whereabouts of horse friends and antagonists as possible distractions. Is there a corner of the yard where your horse is sure that the ghosts hang out? If it's feeding time, you'll probably find her attention elsewhere.

To the degree that you are not able to avoid distractions and less-than-ideal conditions, create a focused, quiet, healing atmosphere within yourself, by staying centered, aware and "in the moment", and project your calm center and confidence to your horse.

The Mental Environment

Thoughts are energy. So are emotions. Our thoughts and emotions create an atmosphere, a mental environment around us at all times, to which horses show great sensitivity.

When you're at your horse's side, or upon her back, your other cares should be elsewhere. If you carry your cares and attitudes with you (and most of us do carry some), leave them outside the paddock gate or outside the barn door or, better yet, down the road miles away. You might start to center and relax yourself on your way to the barn, so that you feel calm and focused when you arrive.

Pamela begins to mentally prepare herself while driving to her horse clients:

> "I empty my mind of all other activity. I deepen my breathing, relax my shoulders and center myself. I bring my attention to the horse. In my mind's eye, I notice if any one area of the horse's body stands out. I mentally talk to the horse, sharing my most loving feelings and admiration for him. I have no expectations or thoughts of goals.
>
> "When I arrive, I ask the horse if I may enter his stall, then do so quietly and respectfully. I kneel near the wall and open my heart to this animal as a partner, as an equal expression of life force. I greet and affirm the intelligence, sensitivity, grace, strength and beauty of the perfect being before me."

Be open and nonjudgemental. Detached from the past and future, observe your horse as she is in this moment, rather than directing your thoughts toward a malfunctioning part or toward results you may hope to achieve — expectations. Thoughts and emotions direct the movement of energy to create events, not necessarily in the form that you really desire. Make no judgements, positive or negative, about yourself or about your horse. Let go of any fears or doubts. "Experience" whatever "is". Trust that you are a catalyst for healing, and let yourself be guided by your horse.

6 *Preparing Yourself*

When you give shiatsu therapy, your body should be relaxed, yet agile and balanced, and your mind calm and focused. In this way, you will be most effective, and aware.

You might already have your own body and/or mind preparation techniques, ones that you have discovered or created that work for you.

The following exercises for stretching and strengthening are ones that Pamela has found useful for her students.

The self-shiatsu techniques are only a few of the many available, and are wonderfully useful for relieving common tensions at any time. There are a number of books that explore this area thoroughly.

Learning to breathe deeply, to move from your center, and to be in the here and now is the pathway towards deeper concentration, towards awareness, towards more fully and truly experiencing life, self and Others, towards joy. The following chapters on these techniques give concepts, insights, images and exercises that we hope you might find helpful.

Stretching and Strengthening Exercises

These exercises are done from a standing position, so they can readily be practised almost anywhere. Sometimes an exercise seems easy when first tried, but produces aching muscles by morning. Take care when trying any unfamiliar exercise. Adjust its degrees and speed to your current muscular condition, and increase gradually from there.

Legs, back, and upper arms
- Stand facing a wall, with your toes 1–2 feet from it, your palms flat against it at shoulder level or just below, and your feet under your hips. Your elbows are soft and slightly bent. Your shoulders are down and relaxed. Your spine is straightly aligned, not arched.
- Let your weight drop down into your heels and forward into your palms, for ten to fifteen seconds. Feel the stretch through the muscles in the back of your legs, from your buttocks to your heels, in your back, and in the back of your upper arms. (These muscle groups are used while riding, as well as for performing shiatsu.)
- Move your feet farther away from the wall 6–8 inches, and repeat.
- Continue to move your feet farther away from the wall in 6–8 inch increments, for as long as you are comfortable, to deepen the stretch. As you move your feet backward, allow your head and shoulders to relax and drop towards the floor. Your back should still be straight, not arched.
- Slowly walk yourself forward to an upright position and drop your arms.

Balance and concentration; lower back and back of thighs

○ Stand with your feet under your hips and your awareness in your center (see "Moving from your center").
○ Focus on a distant point at eye-level.
○ Shift your weight to your right leg; raise your left knee up toward your chest; clasp your hands over your knee and pull it toward your chest for fifteen to thirty seconds.
○ Repeat by changing legs.

Balance; inner and front of thighs

○ Take a very wide stance with your toes pointed outward and your knees aligned with your feet; rest your hands on your thighs.
○ Lower your hips towards the ground by bending your knees, keeping your back straight, and let your hands slide down to your knees and hold there. Your upper body will be slightly bent forward at your waist for balance. Your knees and feet should still be aligned. Hold for three to five seconds.
○ Shift your weight to the right leg as you straighten your left leg; your right heel will raise off the ground. Hold for three to five seconds.
○ Repeat with your weight shifted to the left leg.
○ Recenter your weight and rise up slowly, with your back still straight.

Front of thighs

○ Stand with your back flat against a wall, your pelvis slightly tucked under, your knees slightly bent, and your heels approximately 12–20 inches out from the wall (depending on your height).
○ Slowly slide your flattened back down the wall until your position approximates to that of sitting in a chair. Your arms and hands are relaxed.
○ Hold this position for as long as possible without over-straining your muscles.
○ Slowly slide back up the wall. Depending on your muscular condition, you might want to place two props on either side of you to brace your ascent.

This exercise suits skiers as well as horse therapists and riders.

Relieving Tension with Self-Shiatsu

Shoulders

So many of us seem to hold ourselves up by our shoulders, bracing ourselves to perform a task or solve a problem. The following exercise alone cannot undo years of stress stored in these muscles, but it can help to release some of the tension and pain stored there:

○ Place the fingertips of one hand on top of your opposite shoulder, on the trapezius muscle just above your collar-bone, and press firmly into the muscle. Let your bent elbow drop and relax on your chest.

○ Place the fingers of your other hand in the crease above your elbow and pull your elbow down: you will be pulling your other fingertips into the muscle, and both shoulders down.

○ As you pull down, slowly lower your head away from that muscle towards the opposite shoulder, to stretch it through your neck (Photos 6.1 a–b).

○ Exhale as you pull down your elbow and lower your head.

○ Hold the stretch and pressure for ten seconds or more, then slowly release both.

○ Use your hand to lift your elbow, thereby pushing your other hand to a point farther back on the trapezius muscle. Press your fingertips firmly into the muscle; pull down your elbow with the fingers of your other hand and lower your head toward your opposite shoulder, as you exhale; hold; and slowly release.

○ Again lift your elbow to push your fingertips as far back as possible on the trapezius muscle. Repeat the use of pressure, the stretch through your neck, and the slow release of both.

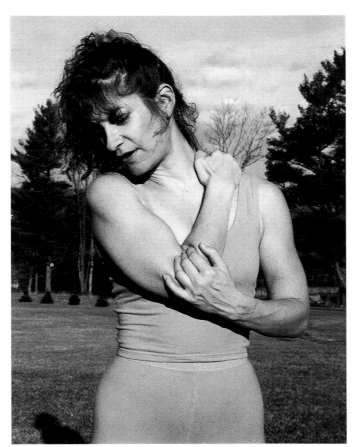

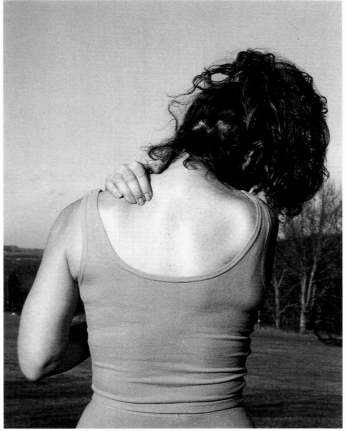

6.1a The fingertips of one hand are pressed into the muscle of the opposite shoulder. The fingertips of the other hand pull the elbow downward through its crease, ...

6.1b ... to increase the firm fingertip pressure on the trapezius muscle. As you pull down on the elbow, lower the head toward the opposite shoulder, so to simultaneously stretch the muscle through the neck.

Hands

○ Press the centre of your palm with the thumb of your other hand. Hold for five to ten seconds. Slowly release.

(This is Point 8 on the Heart Constrictor Meridian. It is known as the "Palace of Anxiety": when we make a fist, that point is stimulated, so we express and relieve anxiety simultaneously. These points are also known in Chinese medicine as the "Palaces of Labour", and considered two of the five main "gates" through which the body's Ki energy communicates with the surrounding environment.)

○ Press the web of your hand, between the thumb and index finger, with the fingertips of the thumb and index finger of your other hand. Hold for five to ten seconds. Slowly release.

(This is Point 4 of the Large Intestine Meridian. It is used to relieve internal irregularities, sinus headaches, infections, and disorders of the lungs and stomach. This point is called the "Great Eliminator".)

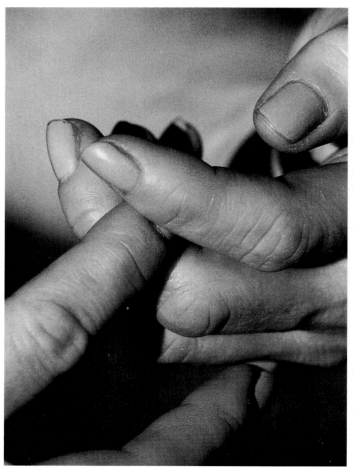

6.2 Pinch the base of each finger with the index and middle finger of the opposite hand. Gently squeeze as you slide them toward the tip, where you squeeze and hold for a moment before continuing to the next finger.

The following exercise stretches and relaxes your fingers, and increases circulation in the hands:

○ Pinch the base of your thumb with two fingers (not fingertips) of your other hand – your thumb and index finger or your index and middle fingers, and, as you squeeze, slide them towards the tip of the thumb. You can stop and hold for a moment at the tip. (See Photo 6.2.)
○ Repeat on each finger of both hands.
○ Shake out your hands.

Breathing

Deep, rhythmic breathing helps you to concentrate, relax, and avoid fatigue. It allows you to fill your lungs to the maximum with life-giving energy, and for that energy to continuously flow. It brings you to your calm center, and helps you to stay there.

Many breathing techniques have been developed by various disciplines, including Yoga, Buddhism and Taoism, for differing goals, but the first goal is for the breath to become calm, natural, smooth, steady and continuous – to enhance health and to calm and focus the mind.

To breathe deeply is to inhale by allowing your diaphragm to descend and your ribs to expand, so your elastic lungs expand fully, so a vacuum is created, and air rushes in. The descending diaphragm, which is dome-shaped when relaxed and flat when contracted, will press upon the contents of the abdomen and cause the front and sides of the abdomen to expand, as well as the lower back. If you place your hands high up on your hips, so that they reach around your waist, they should be pushed outward and "filled" as you inhale, and drawn inward as you exhale. Your rib cage and chest should also gently expand and recede as part of the natural, correct breathing process.

To breathe rhythmically means to give either equal or double time to your exhalations as to your inhalations, continuously, without holding your breath (except in specialized breathing training) or forgetting to breathe. According to Yogic training, the ideal ratio between inhalation and exhalation is 1:2 – in other words, if you inhale for four seconds, you should exhale for eight seconds. Exhalation is emphasized to remove the old air full of gassy wastes, so the fresh air may enter.

Most of us have been told, at some time, to "hold in your stomach and stick out your chest!". I meet people who still carry guilt for disobeying this command. Unfortunately, I see many people carrying pain for obeying it, for it causes an unnatural arch of the back and lots of tense muscles; it poses as "good posture" while it actually destroys it. But I've noticed another thing – that if you hold in your stomach it's very difficult to breathe! It restricts the movement of the chest, and it contracts the abdomen so that the diaphragm can't move, leaving little room for the lungs to expand. If you have learned to carry yourself this way, with your stomach held in and your chest out, the development of deep breathing should bring you a new sense of relaxation, posture and vitality.

Many people, like those who hold in their stomachs and stick out their chests, breathe high, raising their shoulders and collar-bones to let a little air in to the top of the lungs, at the expense of much energy. Other people breathe in the chest, expanding their ribs to fill the mid-section of their lungs, but draw in their abdomens and prevent their diaphragms from functioning. Low breathing depresses the diaphragm, allowing the lower and middle lung regions to fill.

Try to breathe in each of the three regions of your lungs, to become aware of your own breathing habits and of the dynamics and potential of your breathing apparatus:

○ Sit up straight.
○ Contract your abdomen so that your diaphragm can't descend, and breathe in (and out) by raising (and lowering) your shoulders and collar-bones. Take as large a breath as you can.
○ Now, with your abdomen relaxed, expand your chest to let in air (and relax it to exhale). Your abdomen will be sucked in as your chest expands.

Notice, in the two types of breathing, the differences in the use of muscles, tension, and the amount of air you can utilize.

○ Then breathe low by allowing your diaphragm to descend: do not raise your shoulders or chest, but feel with your hands to see that your abdomen is expanding as you inhale and retracting as you exhale.

Compare now the three ways of breathing.

Low breathing utilizes the most air of the three ways, but, to breathe most fully and deeply, you should fill the entire lungs, from the bottom up, allowing your chest to expand as well as your abdomen and lower back, drawing in the maximum amount of air with the minimum of energy. Your shoulders do not help you to breathe, and should be relaxed and down.

If you become aware of the way you breathe, you can learn to deepen your breathing and keep it rhythmic. Breathing exercises develop and strengthen the muscles that are meant to effortlessly facilitate our breathing. They also develop our ability to concentrate and to relax. It's helpful to notice the circumstances under which you shorten your breathing, or forget to breathe. If you can do this, you can change your patterns of response, and possibly the circumstances. You can train yourself to breathe deeply and rhythmically, to relax instead of tense, to focus instead of "freezing up" or "freaking out".

Breathing exercises*
○ Sit comfortably, but erect, with your spine, neck and head aligned.
○ Close the right nostril with your right thumb.
○ Inhale slowly through the left nostril for a count of four seconds.

* Adapted from *The Complete Illustrated Book of Yoga* by Swami Vishnudevananda, Bell Publishing Co. Inc., New York, 1960, pp. 235–7 and pp. 242–3.

○ Try to not make sounds during inhalation. Fill your entire lungs with air, from the bottom up. (I find it helpful to "breathe into my lower back", in order to fully and easily use my diaphragm and rib cage.)
○ Exhale through the same nostril for a count of eight seconds.
○ Repeat this exercise fifteen to twenty times through the left nostril.
○ Close the left nostril, now, with your right ring and little fingers, and remove your thumb.
○ Inhale through the right nostril for four seconds.
○ Exhale through the same nostril for eight seconds.
○ Repeat fifteen to twenty times.

When this exercise feels *very easy* for you, you may increase the proportion of seconds to 5:10, and so on.

Once you feel that you are breathing correctly, automatically, you can progress to the following "alternate breathing" exercise:
○ Close your right nostril with your right thumb.
○ Inhale through the left nostril, for as many seconds as you've become comfortable with.
○ Now, immediately close the left nostril with your right ring and little finger, as you remove your thumb.
○ Exhale through your right nostril, for twice as many seconds as your inhalation. The proportion of inhalations to exhalations is always 1:2.
○ Inhale through your right nostril. Close it with your thumb.
○ Exhale through your left nostril.
○ Repeat this round fifteen to twenty times.

(If you are wondering about the practice of breathing through one nostril, you will probably be interested to know that that is how we normally breathe, by using mostly one nostril for a time, and then the other.)

Your horse's breathing

Your deep, relaxed, rhythmic breathing is a tool to calm your horse, who will hear and feel your calm breath, and possibly imitate it. Breathing audibly can reinforce this aid. Once, as I intently listened to the sounds in Katy's gut and the sensations beneath my hands, I became aware of her audible deep breaths, and realized that I was holding my own breath – my horse was reminding me to breathe.

How we breathe says something about how we feel. For example, a short, sharp inhalation with an audible exhalation (a sigh) seems to indicate a feeling of being overwhelmed, exhausted, defeated. This is as true for horses as for humans. Pamela has developed the technique of mirroring the breathing patterns of her patients, human and horse, in order to understand how they feel, so to help them feel better. You can do this with your horse, to better understand her. While you are dupli-cating her breathing pattern, emotions may become apparent to you. Gradually and audibly deepen your own breathing, perhaps while leaning your body against hers and physically breathing with her – she may now deepen her breathing to match yours.

Moving From Your Center

Our "center" is the balance point within our bodies, and the source of our strength, energy and intuitive movement. In its three dimensions it is our anatomical center of strength. It is known in Chinese medicine as the "Chi (Ki) Ocean", being the main reservoir and source of Ki energy within the body, and the residence of the "Wisdom Mind". The Japanese name for this area is "tan den". It is located within the lower abdomen, centered approximately 1–2 inches below the navel and one to two inches deep within.

All balanced and intuitive movement is initiated from our center. It is from here that natural movement flows. A master swordsman holds his sword with his center; the amateur grips it with his hands. A "horseman" rides from his center, holds the reins with his center, responds and balances from his center, being one with his horse. The greatest effect is achieved, as well as the sense of oneness through touch, when we give shiatsu from our center.

When we move from our center, our attention is focused in the present on our immediate task while our relaxed body performs intuitively. Rather than expending energy through tense muscles in the act of "trying", in the act of passing judgements upon ourselves and/or our activity, we trust and use our body's innate knowledge, we focus our strength and energy to perform our task, we focus and allow it to happen. To move from your center is to move with focused attention and a relaxed body-mind. When we move from our center to give shiatsu, our muscles do not become fatigued. After giving shiatsu treatment from your center, you will find yourself feeling energized, and deeply satisfied, even peaceful.

Moving from your center is a safer, non-stressful, efficient and proficient way to move, while working around your horse, walking through city streets, writing at your desk, holding your morning coffee, brushing your teeth, or in fact performing any activity.

You learn to move from your center with practice, by training your attention. You feel your muscles release their tensions, you breathe low into your abdomen, and you *lower your attention to your center point*. Feel your relaxed and trusting bodymind direct your energy from this area to execute your intentions. Just let it happen.

Exercises
○ Mentally locate your center.
○ Breathe there.

○ Hold a stone with your hands.
○ Now hold it with your center, by moving your awareness from the sensations in your hands and arms to your center. Does the stone feel lighter with your centered awareness?
○ Throw the stone with your center to a designated spot.

○ Stand 20 feet away from a designated location or object.
○ Place your hands, one over the other, over your lower abdomen and

centered about 2 inches below your navel.
○ Walk toward and focus on the designated location or object.
○ Repeat your focused walk, but with your arms relaxed at your sides and your awareness in your center.

Exercise with partner
○ Stand about 10 feet from your partner.
○ Walk towards her, without concentrating on anything in particular, with the intention to pass. As you reach her, your partner will put out one arm to stop you. You will be easily stopped, because you're not paying attention, you are not centered.
○ Now walk by your partner once more, but this time move with your awareness in your center and your attention focused on a destination, a point beyond your standing partner. Direct your energy from your center to this point. Your partner will once again try to stop you with an outstretched arm as you attempt to pass. This time, you will easily pass by, possibly dragging her with you.

Hints
To relax your mind, you must still your mind, by concentration, by "being in the moment".

To relax your body is to release the tensions held in your various muscles. To learn to do this, become aware of the sensation of tension, so that you may know the sensation of a released, relaxed muscle. You might intentionally tense and then release your muscles, one area at a time (your chin, your neck, your right shoulder, upper arm, elbow, lower arm, wrist, hand, a finger, and so on). This exercise is best done when lying flat on your back.

The sensation of tension can be gross or subtle.

As we live, our minds and bodies learn patterns of holding on to tension: knots form in the muscle fibers, restricting movement, our skeletal system becomes misaligned, and our bodies and our movements, as a consequence, become distorted from what is natural, easy and correct. Getting rid of deep-seated tensions and distortions will require more than awareness. It will require time and work, perhaps with one or various practitioners, to gradually release the distortions, and to release old patterns of holding, of movement and of thought. Self-shiatsu, as well as many physical exercises, works to release specific areas.

Each of us learns to hold tension in specific body areas, and carry it there, until we unlearn the habit. If you can identify your body's favorite tension-holding spots, you can direct your attention and your energy to each, one area at a time, and tell your body to release the holding muscles. I know, for instance, that I have an old habit of "holding" myself in the area of my solar plexus: when I notice that sensation, I release the diverted energy held there by letting it "fall" down to my center.

The sensation of moving from your center can give you an addictive high.

Being Here Now

"Concentration is fascination of mind. Where there is love present, the mind is drawn irresistibly toward the object of love. It is effortless and relaxed, not tense and purposeful."

(W. Timothy Gallwey, *The Inner Game of Tennis*,
New York, Random House, 1974, p. 92)

To "be here now" is to be in a relaxed state of awareness. It is the state of bodymind that allows intuitive thought and action to flow, that lets you "go beyond yourself", and "everything to fall into place". When "here now", your consciousness is fully absorbed in the present moment, no thought-tendrils reaching to the past or future. You trustingly allow your mental barriers to fall away, open yourself to the universe, and allow the knowledge that's there to flow through you.

What prevents you from "being here now"? An active ego, a need for control, a judgemental mind, and the positive and negative expectations that we habitually ponder. Mostly, we lack the trust to allow ourselves to experience and respond to the present moment without actively "doing" something.

In his *Letters To a Young Poet*, Rainer Maria Rilke explains that the artist's "clarity" is found when one is:

"... not reckoning and counting, but ripening like the tree which does not force its sap and stands confident in the storms of spring without the fear that after them may come no summer. It does come. But it comes only to the patient, who are there as though eternity lay before them, so unconcernedly still and wide."

(Letter No. 3, April 23, 1903, translated by M. D. Herter
Norton, W.W. Norton & Co., New York, 1954, p. 30.)

You enter the "here and now" by stilling your mind, by focusing it on something in present time. There are no "if only's" or "should be's" or "maybe if's". The only verb tense is the present: I am, s/he is, it is, we are, you are, they are. You do not "try" to focus your mind; you just let it focus, by allowing it to become absorbed, "fascinated". As you become one with your activity or with the object of your focus, your mind lets go of its chatter. You enter the calm in your center. Your mind clears to sense what is actually happening, and you take appropriate action.

I've found the ease and joy of being in the "here and now", while standing by my mare on a crystal winter morning, hearing the rhythmic crush of grain within her jaws, seeing the dawning sun in ice doilies on the glass, feeling her warm nearness. I've found it while cleaning her stall, fully absorbed in finding clumps of dark manure and wet shavings. I've found it on a long show-day afternoon, cantering a course, hearing, feeling, jumping in the perfect cadence of her stride.

To stay "in the moment", when giving shiatsu, listen for the energy. Feel it. Feel it from your center. Feel its movement, as it pulsates, stagnates, slows, rushes. Focus on its presence, absence, nature and flow, and your attention will be in the "now", moment to moment, pulse to pulse, stillness to pulsation.

An exercise to focus your attention here, now, is to watch your breath. Watch it go in, then out, and in, and out, of your nose or your mouth. Watching your breath with full concentration will immediately bring you to your calm center and keep you "in the moment".

Once you have experienced "being here now", you can and will expand that experience through a growing trust, a trust in releasing the mind from the responsibility and need to control. You'll find a joy in just "being", in letting go, in trust. Joy is addictive.

"Being here now" is the safest and sanest place to be, where clarity of sense and action flows out of a calm center.

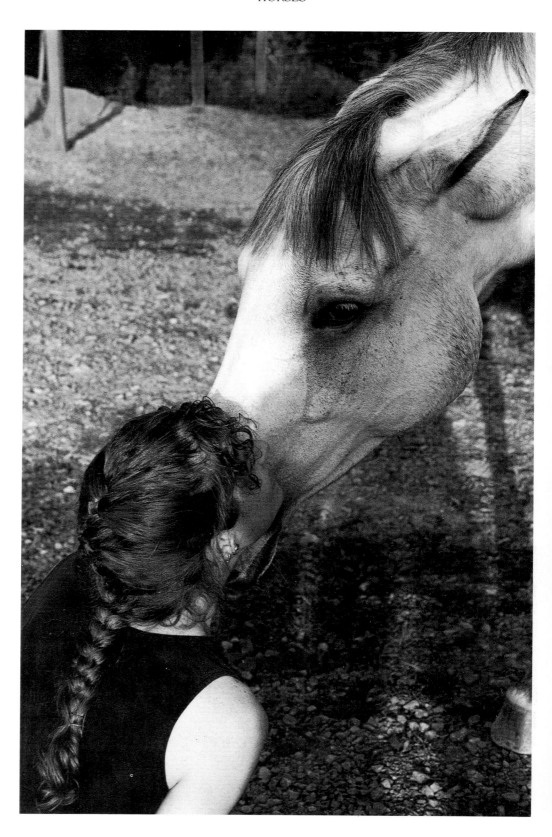

Listen.

7 *Evaluating Problems*

"The only thing necessary is to see, to hear, to ask, and to feel what the bodymind of the person is saying."

(Dianne M. Connelly, PhD, M. Ac., *Traditional Acupuncture: The Law of the Five Elements*, The Center for Traditional Acupuncture, Colombia, MD, p. 107.)

Talking Horse

Horses continuously express what is happening physically and emotionally within them. It is up to us, as their friends and caretakers, to become receptive to their modes of speech, to learn to understand what they would tell us and do tell us, to listen and "hear" them, and their needs.

We need to "talk Horse". We need to talk with the full, true and dictionary meaning of "talk", which is to communicate or exchange thoughts, feelings or desires. To "talk", to exchange with another, requires one to "listen". How do you listen to a horse? With your eyes, your sensing hands, your entire body, your intuitive perception, with no prejudgements, with your mind open, clear and focused, with your attention centered. Horses, excepting the walled-off mind of the abused, possess a sensitive understanding of human intentions and state of mind; they "speak" to receptive minds and eyes.

Listening to Body Language

Horses talk with their bodies. Their words are shaped by a tilt of an ear,

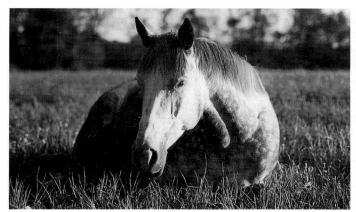

7.1a *Katydid had jumped the fence and eaten too much rich spring grass. I knew by her facial expressions and by her occasional glance at her abdomen that she was feeling intestinal discomfort, not having a rest. I used pressure on the points for indigestion/colic, and here I'm giving her a few quiet moments before I ask her to stand and walk.*

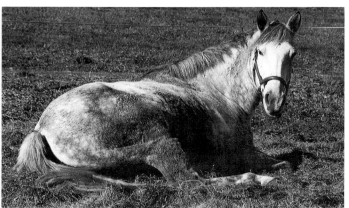

7.1b *Sunbathing. Note the different expression of her eyes and body language from the preceding photograph: her demeanor is relaxed, alert to her surroundings, not stressed.*

a thrust of neck, a turn of quarters, a shake of withers, a hoof treading air, or appearing glued, as a post, to the ground. The human eye learns to "see" what is physically and gesturally "normal" for the individual, and then may discern deviations and changes. The educated eye becomes increasingly aware of and respondent to subtle physical and behavioral nuances, and can so avoid potential problems. Awareness of a horse's individual personality and history can help to guide your intuitive and empirical comprehension of her gestures. (See Photos 7.1a–b.)

In a physical conversation with your horse, she might push towards you a sore or needy body area, present you with an injured limb, or pull a limb or area away from you to protect it from further pain. You would respond with observing eyes and an understanding tone of voice and gestures, exploring the limb or area with feeling hands, or beginning your touch in a comfortable and welcomed zone as you gain her trust and the release of tensions and fear.

A horse may show that you've touched pain by flinching and twitching her muscles, tucking her tail under, staring coldly with wide or narrowed eyes, flattening her ears, showing aggression, or moving away.

The release of tension and pain can generate a horse's response of chewing, licking, yawning, a lowering of the head (signifying trust), a relieved sigh, a hug, and large grateful eyes. Their eyes may express surprise, from a new awareness, sensation or flexibility. The expression of their eyes and ears may tell you that you've found the needy point or area, that you should continue to hold or press where you are. Other body gestures may say the same.

> After a roll in the mud, Kate presented me with her hind end. Was her tail itchy? – or did she want a point pressed. I didn't know, but started by scratching her dock, then moved a sensing and pressing thumb down the Bladder Meridian of the buttocks. As soon as I pressed on the Point of Buttock, she moved her tail aside and over my hand, firmly pressing and holding my thumb in place. This, she made quite clear, was what she wanted.

Body gestures and facial expressions will also tell you to "bug off", that if you persist with what you are doing, you may be nipped, kicked or swatted. You may see flattened ears, anguished or narrowed eyes, a protruding lip, or, perhaps, a flailing and retracted leg. The area, a memory, or your technique may be too painful, or the area may not be in need. You learn to discern the differences. If the gestural motivation is pain, you should move to an area where your horse enjoys being touched before carefully reapproaching the painful one. As you continue to work with your horse, you continue to monitor her responses and to adjust yours accordingly.

The memory of pain and mental pain can readily produce symptomatic habits in horses, as well as in people. Long after the real pain and its cause have vanished, the memory will remain until the horse (or person)

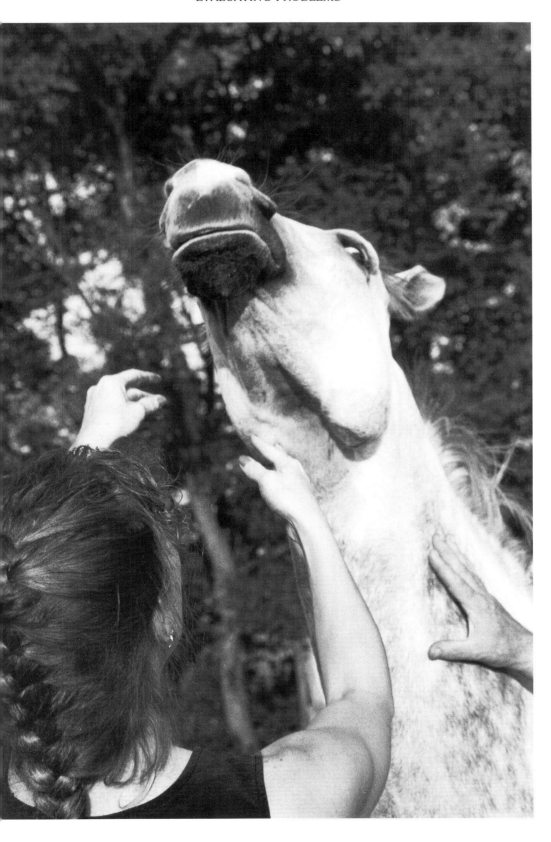

Our temperamental model demands a break.

is made awares, on a sensory level, that the pain and its cause and consequences no longer exist. A horse may not have regained former flexibility merely because she hasn't regained awareness of, or belief in, that bodily potential. If the pain is mental, and fear is present, you must, beyond removing a cause, re-establish trust and confidence. A horse is likely to be more sensitive and reactive to the memory of pain and to mental pain than to "real", present physical pain. Such pain should be approached, diagnosed and treated with all the more consideration and respect for the emotions and time that have held that pain in place. Replacing pain and fear with pleasure and trust is essential to treatment. Recognizing, and understanding, the nature of this pain is essential to its diagnosis. (See TECHNIQUES: Touching Pain, p. 73.)

Listening Through Your Body

Your horse listens to your body when you ride, to your touch when you groom, to the quality in your voice when you speak, to your mind when you are present. The "horseman" listens to his horse through the same channels, conversing, responding.

Riding

The good rider rides with "feel", in continuous conversation with his horse. When you ride with feel, you note even the faintest sign that your horse may have a problem. Once dismounted, you observe with your eyes and palpate with your hands (if possible, have someone walk and trot your horse for you, or use a lunge line). You allow your hands to work intuitively, perhaps "illogically". Your hands sense the presence of heat, energy blocks, imbalances, while you work to correct them and observe her responses. (If the signs warrant it, you of course take monitoring tests, such as temperature and pulse, and consult your veterinarian and/or farrier.) Some horses are so willing to do their work that they will compensate for any soreness, effectively disguising it in order to perform, until cumulative and compounded aggravation becomes a debilitating injury. (See SOME DEFINITIONS: Source Versus Symptoms, p. 10.) With such willing horses you must be particularly alert and sensitive to even the vaguest lessening of performance.

Grooming

You groom your horse with feel. Note where your horse shows sensitivity and explore if it's a response to soreness, memory, or an insensitive grooming technique. Adjust your pressure, speed and stroke to your horse's response. Work intuitively, allowing your curry comb or brush to be drawn in to give deep, massaging pressure, and to lighten, slow and caress where it seems to want to, confirming or adjusting your pressure and technique by your horse's response. Groom your horse as you yourself would like to be stroked and pressed and scratched, losing the boundary between her skin and yours. Let your grooming tool become part of your hand, and your hand the tool when it seems appropriate.

Through aware grooming, you grow to know your horse's body, her particular sensitivities, her comfortable zones, her itchy spots and her muscular condition. You notice changes, and can respond immediately to treat signs of soreness or injury as part of your grooming ritual. Intuitive pressing or massaging with your curry comb or brush may be enough to eliminate an energy blockage or loosen tightened muscle fibers.

Your "routine" should be as flexible as your responses to your horse, to the present state of her bodymind. A lengthened grooming session may shorten or eliminate your ride for that day, but can grant you days, weeks or months of rides otherwise lost to your horse's resistance, lessened performance, or injury.

Imitating
Pamela has discovered an extremely effective technique for "listening" to a horse's body through her own, a way of diagnosing by imitation and recreation of the physical sensations:

> "When diagnosing a horse, I always want, if possible, to see him move at the walk and trot. After first observing him, I often move behind him, and imitate his movement as much as possible considering my physical limitations. I move my hips the same way, my legs, and feet. I even mimic his head movement. This creates a feeling for the way he uses his energy or doesn't use it. Of course, the front of the body is more difficult to mimic, but it is possible, through centered concentration, to get a clear feeling for this as well. After a short time it is possible to really feel, from the inside out, the action and reaction of imbalances, facilitating diagnosis.

> "Some people are so sensitive, they may actually experience physical pain where the horse does. I don't encourage this type of transference, as it can be exhausting, if not downright unhealthy.

> "When learning this technique, first walk behind a horse who seems to move in a balanced way. Then walk behind one who does not, and compare the feelings. Don't forget to breathe. Sometimes, while doing this, I quiet my breathing and make it very shallow, in order to be conscious only of the other individual, and not of myself."

Listening to Intuition, Inner Sight and Speech

Intuitive knowledge is our truest, deepest knowledge. When we quiet the mind and open it wide, we may hear the voice of the universe, our inner voice, and the voice of those who lack verbal speech. Countless people speak of receiving thought-transference from their animals. I believe, when my horses demonstrate a thorough understanding of complex verbal dialogue, that it is through thought, or mental image transference, rather than a grasp of English grammar and vocabulary. It is as though, through a mutual desire to communicate, our word-thoughts are transposed into a form intelligible to the other.

To receive intuitive knowledge, inner sight and speech, you must be receptive to it, welcome it, acknowledge it, trust it. As you learn to recognize and acknowledge it, you notice that it comes more often. "Listen" to it. This may take practice, with the shedding of learned doubt. But, always, "listen" to it.

Pamela works intuitively. She feels it is the only correct method. Given this premise, and trusting it fully, she has access to invaluable, enriching knowledge to guide her.

"My work with the horse begins before actual contact is made. When having a conversation on the telephone with the horse owner or caretaker, I open myself up to any and all impressions. By this I mean that I am relaxed yet alert, and often I will see an image of a certain area of the animal's body, not necessarily the area that the person is speaking of. By trusting my instincts, I find that I may be tuning in to another area that is in stress, perhaps the original injury, that is causing a series of compensation problems.

"When I greet the horse, I may invite him to share with me whatever he likes, be it some emotional pain or physical. Sometimes I am flooded by an emotion, like grief, frustration, loneliness. By being confident that I am in my center, I know that these feelings are coming from the horse.

"After a short time, I am given 'permission' to begin: a nuzzle, a nudge, a deep sigh (to me, a sure sign that we have made mental contact). I stand and, with relaxed eyes, scan the body. My eyes may be drawn to certain areas, or linger someplace. I feel that these may be problem areas, to be approached gently and after working on more comfortable areas first.

"After working only a few minutes, and at intervals throughout the session, I may ask to see the horse move, unless he's in too much pain. By the relaxed eye method, I can continue to see how he's using or not using his body, his energy."

When you work in an intuitive, trusting way, you may be surprised to find your hands drawn to an area seemingly unrelated to a symptomatic one. Do not judge. Follow your intuitive sense. It is very likely that you have found the source of a series of compensation problems, of an old injury, of an undetected injury.

Kate gave an occasional hint of being "off" at the trot, and she bucked and coughed the twice I asked for a left-lead canter. These were my only clues. That evening in her stall, I placed my palms on points by the hip socket. She stepped away from my touch. "All right," I said, "I'll let you be." I noticed that she had moved her right shoulder toward me, but I turned to leave. As I did, I felt a pain in my own right shoulder. I, gratefully, understood, and placed my hands now where intuition, not mind, led them, to her shoulder and elbow. The next day she moved without a problem or resistance.

The point is not that I received and recognized a psychic transference of pain, but that I stayed receptive. I accepted my mistake in attempting to treat Kate's hip, and "heard" her movements as part of our conversation, rather than as resistance (a negative declaration). I stayed open to be guided by my intuition and my horse, rather than by my analytical or sceptical mind.

Listening Through Touch: Diagnosing Energy Imbalances

The circumstances of the moment, your horse and your intuition will dictate how you will proceed. You might move your sensing palm or fingers along the Bladder Meridian, to sense the quality and quantity of the energy flow. The Bladder Meridian is a good indicator of the general state of health of the horse. As you feel the energy or its lack, you simultaneously work to correct imbalances. (See SHIATSU TREATMENT: A Shiatsu Massage: Diagnosis and Treatment, p. 89.) You might rest your relaxed eyes upon your horse and see if your nonjudgemental attention is drawn to any particular areas, then confirm, adjust and further diagnose through touch. If an area is not overly sensitive, you work to correct imbalances as you sense them. You might proceed by allowing your hands to be drawn to and work where they seem to "want to go" on your horse's body. My horse, Katydid, has gained through shiatsu treatment such awareness of her body that I can verbally ask if she needs my help as I present her with my raised, open palms: if she is wanting, she moves the appropriate body areas into my palms for me to proceed with treatment. Once you are more adept at sensing the Ki energy, you will seek to locate the areas of kyo and jitsu — and bring them into balance.

As you work, observe passively, and allow your hands to be as catalysts for the healing process. Allow yourself, through your hands, to be drawn into your horse's body, as you stay centered, relaxed, fully focused in the moment, aware of the sensations, reactions and responses that you receive. Allow oneness to happen between you, as a portal to the state and needs of her bodymind. It is important for you to stay as clear and centered as possible, so that you will not confuse your own sensations, sentiments or prejudgements with the information received from your horse.

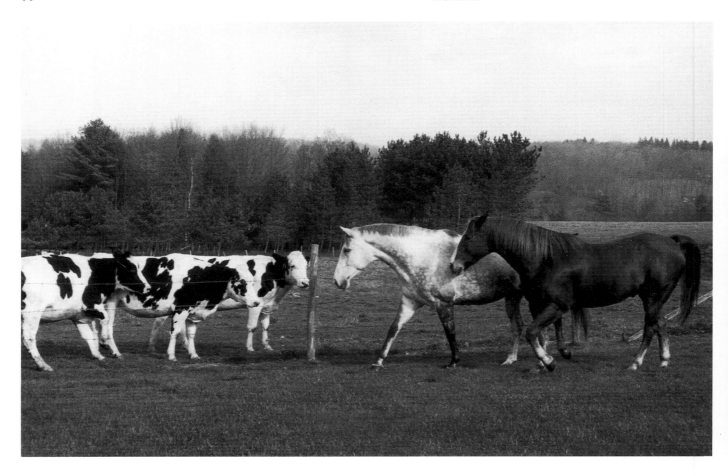

"Do you speak Horse?"

Seeing Wholeness

When evaluating your horse's problems, remember that she is a body-mindspirit functioning as a whole, integrated unit, not as a collection of parts. Any incapacitation of one part will muster aid from the rest of the body in the attempt to restore balance, causing the spread and cumulative effects of stress. Symptoms travel down from up and up from down and diagonally. By the time a symptom is evident, it may appear physically distant from its originating cause. The source of unexplained lameness is often found above, and lower back pain can emanate from the opposing shoulder or the foot. Too often, the symptom receives treatment, but not the silent, invisible persisting cause. Your horse and your inner sight are often more likely to find this cause than is your analytical mind.

Diagnosing External Causes

Be alert to potential external causes of your horse's physical problems. An ill-fitting saddle is a common one, as is rider imbalance and stiffness. Among other possibilities are an inappropriate bit, improperly used training devices, improper shoeing, nutritive deficiencies, insufficient bedding, toxic plants in the paddock, lack of companionship, stressful "companionship", or lack of exercise. Perhaps your horse is, after all, not ideally suited for the work you ask of her, either physically or mentally. Or perhaps her/your training program needs to backtrack to basics and rebuild muscle conditioning, flexibility and confidence. Hopefully you have a veterinarian, farrier and trainer/competent observer who could aid you in any such investigations. It will be of little use to relieve your horse's symptoms if the cause remains to chronically reproduce them.

8 *Feeling Energy*

Our fingertips are filled with nerves to facilitate our sense of touch, our "feel" of the world. And yet, each of us would describe the same sensation in different terms, filtered through our own experience, through our unique bodymindspirit.

Some of the terms shiatsu practitioners use to describe how energy feels to their touch are: a tingling, like tiny sparks, subtle to gross vibrations, subtle and faint pulsations, an echo, a bubbling, a feeling of something pushing up under and toward your touch.

Learning to "feel" energy is actually quite simple. It only requires you to relax, focus, and gradually tune your awareness to the sensations that are there. This means that you must, at least momentarily, give up the mental clutter and clatter that distracts us all, that you must turn your attention to your receiving hands and the energy system that they are listening to.

You listen in a relaxed state, ready to receive whatever comes. Have no prejudgements about your ability, nor about what is there to be felt. Have no expectations that you "will" feel, nor of what you may feel. Simply do it with awareness, and a new awareness will come.

I believe that we all feel energy through our touch, but that, for many of us, our awareness of the feeling is blocked. It is blocked by tensions and distractions. There is too much noise, of the mental, emotional and physical sort, around us. Some of us live with an aware sense of the energetic life force, Ki, and its communicative properties. However, for most of us, it is time, patience, and trust that allows this sense to develop.

Time and practice increase one's awareness, not only of the energy flow, but of the subtleties within it, and even of the quantity and quality within each pulsation. The differences within the flow are often barely perceptible, but, with practice, your ability to sense and recognize them will become more and more refined.

At first, you will want to recognize a sensation of energy pulsing, flowing. What you feel might fit one of the descriptive phrases given in the beginning of this chapter. You may also be able to sense regions of heat or cold. A full-blown inflammation has obvious heat, but tight muscle tissue, jitsu areas, give off varying degrees of heat. Jitsu areas, that block and accumulate energy, may feel tight, hard where it should not be;* they may feel raised, or "full"; they may actually vibrate with an overdose of energy, subtly or visibly. Remember that jitsu is mostly Yang, and that Yang is active and obvious, as the rays of the sun on a clear day, or an uninhibited boy at play. The kyo areas, which are mostly Yin, are deprived of energy. They may feel silent, still, "empty"

* Obviously bone is hard; and the neck ligament that runs from the poll to the withers does and should feel hard.

or "hollow", maybe "concave", sometimes cold; they are quiet and inward; their need is the source of problems, of symptoms. It is easier to find and identify jitsu areas.

If you are not already intimately familiar with your horse's body, with her muscle tone and her range and manner of movement, you may now become so. As your hands explore her body for sensations of energy, be aware of how the various muscle groups feel: in the hindquarters, the shoulder, the neck, along the back. Then begin to differentiate between the condition of the muscles within each group (refer to the diagrams of the muscle groups in each treatment chapter). Notice where the muscles feel hard and tight (and the position of her body: if she's contracting the muscle, as for support when one hind leg is fully weighted, or for bend as in the neck, the muscle should feel tight). Healthy muscles feel supple and resilient. Healthy muscles also look supple and resilient when they move. Train your eyes and your hands to assess your horse's condition, and you will learn to eliminate problems before serious symptoms appear.

As you use the shiatsu technique of pressure to treat your horse, notice what you feel or don't feel. Merely observe the sensations or lack of them as you work. Do this also when you are grooming, tacking up, riding, or just being around your horse:

○ Lay your relaxed (not limp) hand upon her and note any sensations.
○ If you feel nothing, don't judge, don't become impatient or discouraged, don't "give up". It's possible that your horse's energy is balanced where you have touched her, and so there is nothing dramatic for you to feel. It's also possible that you placed your hand on a kyo area, low in energy at that moment, or on an area where a major meridian is not running close to the surface.
○ Move your hand to try in another area.
○ Try gradually leaning a little of your weight into your hand – it sometimes intensifies the sensations.
○ Try holding your hand just off your horse's body, so that you barely feel the hairs, and see if you feel any sensations of heat, or cold, of tightness, or "emptiness", of energetic activity, or of none. If you are aware of sensations, focus on them as you very slowly move your relaxed hand away from your horse's body, noting at what point the sensations fade (Photo 8.1).

  (The ability of some people to feel energy off the body is not a needed skill, though it's one that you could develop with practice. You should certainly not doubt yourself for a lack of it. It is only mentioned as an exercise useful in focusing your attention and sensibility.)

You may doubt what you feel. This is normal when you are learning a new skill, especially one that is not observable and confirmable by someone's eyes. You may think that it is your own energy, or pulse, that you are feeling. If you do think this, try resting your relaxed fingertips on various parts of your own body, and note the subtle differences in the

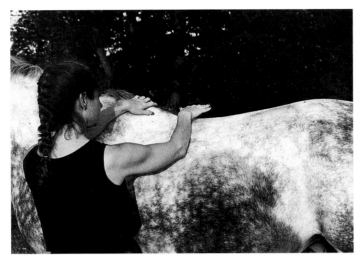

8.1 *With her supporting hand resting on the withers, Pamela very slowly moves an open, relaxed, sensing palm over the Bladder Meridian and the muscles of the back and hindquarters. Her palm is two to three inches from the body. She is noting any sensations that meet her palm, such as heat, coolness, a faint pull or push, tingling or itchiness.*

sensations. Do the same on an agreeable friend's body. And now on inanimate objects. If you were merely feeling the energy or pulse in your own fingertips, everything would feel the same to you.

Your horse can feel you and your intentions very clearly. Your touch affects her, whether you sense it happening or not. Confirmation of this truth will be in the changes that you will see, some immediately, others over time. These changes, "results", can take the form of a calmer disposition, a more willing and responsive temperament. They can be relaxed muscles giving improved, fuller performance. "Results" can be the disappearance of an "odd" or unexplained symptom or habit, such as a cough, head tossing, head shyness, being occasionally or chronically "off", or flattened ears every time you appear with the saddle. You may also notice changes in yourself, perhaps a greater calm, an ability to focus your attention, to give yourself over to the moment, to whatever you are doing. You may have more patience. Very likely, your ability to "listen" and "hear" and "see" will be enhanced. And you will learn to speak to your horse through your touch.

Exercise
○ Sit straight up in a chair or on the floor. Relax your shoulders. Shake out your hands to relax them. Take deep, full breaths, and continue to do so throughout the exercise. Hold your hands at chest level with the fingers straight but relaxed, with no tension in them, and the palms facing each other several inches apart.
○ Notice any sensations, such as a pulling together or a pushing away, heat or cold.

○ Bring your palms closer together without touching, and then again apart, noting the increase and decrease in sensations.
○ See how far apart you can move your palms and still sense some activity.

Exercise with partner
○ Stand behind your partner, who is sitting in a chair.
○ Close your eyes, shake out your hands, breathe deeply.
○ Slowly bring your palms toward your partner's shoulders.
○ Be aware of any sensations, such as of heat, coldness, being pulled in, or of energy pushing up toward you.
   One shoulder will often give more information than the other: the side with more tension may feel hotter, and seem to pull your hand toward it out of need, or push your hand away, being too full of painful muscle spasm to yet tolerate being touched.
○ Bring your hands closer still. Now lay relaxed palms on top of your partner's shoulders and gently hold them there.
○ Again, be aware of any sensations that you receive.
○ Describe what you feel to your partner, who should in turn tell you what he feels is happening in his shoulders (tense, tight, achy, warm, cold, relaxed, and so on). He should also tell you how your touch feels to him.

You shouldn't worry if you don't feel very much in the beginning. Perhaps you need to be more relaxed, to breathe more deeply, or time and practice to tune your sensory awareness. And/or perhaps your partner needs to relax more.

○ Next, using the heels of your palms, with your fingers resting relaxed upon the shoulder, exert gradual, gentle pressure on the top of your partner's shoulder muscles (be sure that you are not pressing on bone).
○ Notice if one side feels stiffer, more or less resistant to your touch.
○ Now, on one shoulder, use your thumb to gently press in the same area, while your palm lays resting on the other side. Alternate, to use thumb pressure on the other side.
○ Once again, lay your relaxed hands on your partner's shoulders and note the sensations, as you did in the beginning of this exercise.
○ Slowly lift your hands off, as you notice if you still feel some kind of contact. Are the "off-the-body" sensations somehow changed?
○ Discuss with your partner the sensations that you both have felt.

Switch positions with your partner, so that you both have the experience of trying to feel energy through your hands, and of being touched in this way. You should both receive and use the feedback on how your touch feels to the other person. Perhaps you need to relax your hands more, or make them more "there", less limp. Perhaps you are pressing too hard, or not firmly enough. Your horse will tell you in her own language.

How your touch is perceived has as much to do with the person or horse receiving it, as with yourself: a thoroughbred generally has more sensitive skin than many other breeds; the muscles of some people and horses are so tight and sore that the lightest touch can make them scream; and there are people and horses who have learned to defend themselves with a callous coating, dulling their senses to not feel pain. As you learn to feel energy, you will also tune your awareness to the other being you are working with, so that you will adjust your touch to their need of that moment.

9 *Moving Energy*

Ki flowing freely through the meridians regulates and balances the molecular and cellular systems. Energy blocks create imbalance and, eventually, dis-ease. Shiatsu techniques release the energy so it may flow and restore balance/health.

Shiatsu reaches deep muscles and moves vertebrae by informing or releasing the Ki energy to do so. Movement of energy will release tightened muscles so that bones may be eased back into place. Sending energy to a muscle attachment, where spasms originate, can allow spontaneous structural adjustments. Techniques of stretching a meridian and rotating and stretching joints also allow muscles to relax and energy to flow.

The techniques employed to move energy are: two-point pressure, rotation, stretching, "jiggling", percussion, and moving muscle.

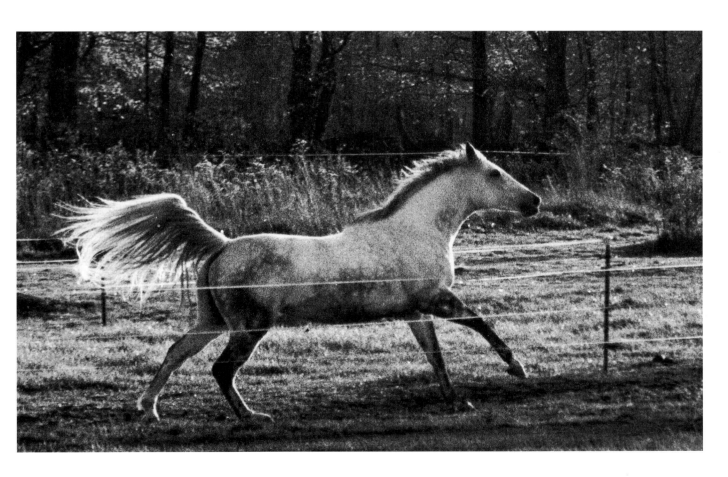

A Supporting Hand, A Moving Hand

Shiatsu is applied by giving two-point pressure: one to support as the other moves energy. We therefore speak of a **supporting** hand and a **moving** hand. The pressures are variably applied by the palm, the fingers, the thumb, the blade of hand, the elbow and the arm, depending on the type of pressure or degree of sensitivity needed. Whatever part of the hand or body is applied, there is always one pressure to support and a second to stimulate the movement of energy. This provides YinYang balance of pressure, so to stimulate a balanced energy flow.

The supporting hand is a quiet, stabilizing force. It "tonifies"*, it brings warmth. It has the quality of Yin. The moving hand is the actively working hand. It has the quality of Yang.

The supporting hand silently performs essential tasks. It firstly provides the warm, soothing, supportive quality of a quiet hand, relaxing the body to receive treatment. It distracts pain when the moving hand contacts a sensitive point. It senses the movement of energy, and which way it wants to move to find balance. When it holds a leg joint, it senses the range of motion and changes in the energy and motion range, while supporting the horse to release tension. It gives support and a sense of balance to the practitioner. And it completes a circle of oneness between the energy of the practitioner and that of the patient.

The moving hand actively pushes, pulls, stimulates, shakes up, relaxes, sedates, and confirms the presence of the energy.

Pressure

You give pressure from your center, in a relaxed state. You should give it without tension, especially in your mind, hands, arms and shoulders. The degree of strength needed will come from your center and through your arms, not from your wrist, palm or fingers, and not from "trying to press". Focus, from your center, on the sensations beneath your touch and your horse's response, rather than on your hand, elbow or arm.

Degree: natural and supportive
There is a misconception that effective shiatsu requires deep, hard, painful pressure. The contrary is true. In Japan, in recent centuries, a form of acupressure massage developed that utilized the deep-pressure technique to effect the relaxation and pleasure of the client, rather than, as shiatsu, the restoration of health. Deep pressure, which is sedating, does not by itself rebalance the energy; it does not deal with the originating cause of symptoms; and it can worsen disease.

Deep pressure can further deplete the low store of energy of Yin/kyo-type patients. A shiatsu session should produce dynamic relaxation, not tiredness. Deep pressure can increase blockage, calling in more energy and compounding a Yang/jitsu condition (such as inflammation). Prolonged deep pressure will close off meridians, creating new dams. And deep pressure can feel painful. Pain causes a person or horse to tense,

*"Tonification" is the shiatsu technique for treating kyo (weak, depleted) areas. The technique sends warmth deep within the body to nurture strength and normalization. The term derives from the physiological meaning of "tone", which is "the natural firmness of the tissues and normal functioning of bodily organs in health" (*Collins English Dictionary*).

to close themselves protectively, rather than to relax and open themselves for the smooth flow of energy.

Natural, gentle, supportive pressure will bring the deepest, greatest effect. You may gauge your pressure by what feels good, natural and comfortable to you, without an exertion of "effort". See yourself as a catalyst that stimulates healing through your touch, rather than as a healing force. You are having a conversation, not giving a lecture.

> When I turn my mare to a fence, my seat and legs say "Yes," through her sides, "continue your rhythm and stride up to the fence and over to the other side." Mostly she responds, "Great! Let's go." But some days she queries back, "Are you sure? You want me to jump **that**?" "Yes!" I say with increased pressure. If I press insensitively, too hard, she'll move off away from my legs, speed tensely from my touch, and break our circle of energy.

Gauge your degree of pressure to your horse's needs of the moment, to her sensitivity and temperament, and to where you are pressing. Arabians and Thoroughbreds are generally thin-skinned and sensitive, while a heavily muscled Quarter Horse may require more pressure, and a thick-furred pony a bit more. Heavily muscled areas will take more pressure than will bony ones.

Deeper pressure may be needed to reach through and under heavily muscled areas or tightened muscles, but should be gradually, sensitively applied, then quickly released. This may be repeated a few times, if needed, in the same location.

Your response should be intuitive, directed by your horse's need – the need in that moment, in that specific spot. How deep, how long and where you press is not dictated by what you "think", but rather by what "feels right".

Time to hold: 2–30 seconds
It is essential to hold patiently, without movement and without expectations. Steady pressure penetrates into the body and activates energy, stimulates the parasympathetic nervous system, calms the internal organs, and effects the body as a whole. Pressure may be held for two seconds to thirty seconds. Two seconds may be sufficient, or longer may be needed to feel some response from the energy flow. If you hold for up to thirty seconds and feel no change, move on to the next point or area and return to this point later in the session. You may then find the condition changed, either from your further treatment in other areas or from a prolonged response.

Direction: vertical
The most precise and effective pressure is given at a ninety-degree angle, that is vertically, perpendicularly, to the skin surface. Vertical pressure goes to the base of the tsubo and fills it.

Palm pressure

The palm gives a softer, less penetrating pressure. It is supportive. It brings warmth to the area, to prepare it for treatment, to release tension, and to "tonify" (see footnote on p. 52). (At the center of your palms are the points (HC #8) which, in Chinese medicine, are considered two of the five "gates" through which the body's Ki energy senses and communicates with the surrounding environment.)

Your hand, your palm and fingers, should relax and mold to the body's contour. Be sure not to hold tension in your fingers. As your relaxed hand rests on your horse's body, you send pressure through your arm into the heel of your palm. As pressure increases, your wrist bends, while the curve of elbow stays soft and your shoulders relaxed.

You gradually increase pressure, for two or three seconds maybe, hold for what feels like the appropriate time, and gradually release. Many people tend, at first, to release abruptly, but it's important to release slowly.

Fingertip pressure

The fingertips are used for more penetrating and specific work, and, with their concentration of nerve endings, to more sensitively feel energy, or the lack of it.

With a relaxed thumb, your four fingers touch and softly curve to form a linear unit of the tips. The unit presses along the meridian lines and the muscle fibers, rather than across them. Most of the pressure is given through your center fingers, but it's more comfortable to use the four as a unit. If your fingernails aren't short, flatten the tips to prevent the nails from digging in as you press. The heel of the palm of your same hand can rest on your horse, for her comfort and yours.

Pressure is gradually applied, held, then gradually withdrawn. For some areas above your shoulder height, such as the Bladder Meridian next to the spine, you will need to use a pulling-down pressure to achieve a ninety-degree angle (as always, comfortably, without strain, from your center). (See Photo 9.1.)

Thumb pressure

Thumb pressure is the most specific. It is also a sensitive sensing tool. It can be too intense to use extensively on horses, so we use it, lightly, on smaller bony areas, like the face and legs, and we use it to apply very specific, deeply penetrating pressure to points. You would use thumb pressure on colic points in an emergency, or to reach through heavy, tight muscles. When comfortable for the patient and practitioner, it is used to give point-to-point technique, to send the body the clearest messages. (See Photo 9.2.)

Just the tip or the entire pad of the thumb may be used, depending on where you are pressing and the degree applied. While working along a meridian with your thumb as the "moving" pressure, you may sometimes apply your other thumb as the "supporting" pressure, to give very specific warmth and comfort as it "listens" for a response.

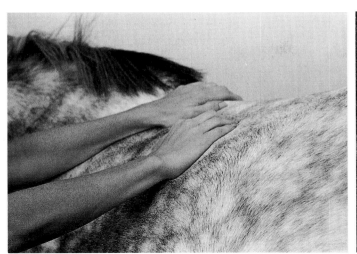

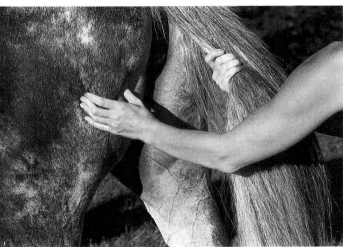

9.1 Fingertip pressure. The nearby supporting hand gives gentle, total contact from the wrist to the fingertips. The moving hand is slightly cupped so that the four fingertips are aligned and in contact with the horse's skin, so to drop pressure vertically inward. The heel and thumb of this hand rest upon the horse. The two hands and the horse become one.

9.2 Thumb pressure on deep muscle. Pamela is using a slight push pull technique: she is leaning her weight into her thumb and bent front leg as she holds the tail (bone) firmly and counterweights her back foot. She gives deeper pressure without strain (notice that her arm is relaxed). Her thumb is positioned along the Bladder Meridian at the hamstring muscle, which can take, and often wants, such pressure.

Hand-blade pressure

The hand blade can be used to smash wood or to heal the body. For healing, we use a slightly curved hand, and any edge of it. It is used on the shoulder area, to press beneath the shoulder-blade and the shoulder muscles (see Photos 18.19a–f and 18.20a–f in SHIATSU TREATMENT: The Shoulders and Forelegs, pp. 128 & 130). You place the hand on the desired location and gradually lean weight into it, increasing the pressure. If your horse will accept deeper pressure, continue to lean in. You can use lower-body strength, and avoid strain, by resting the elbow of your working hand against your hip area. As always, you hold, then release slowly.

Elbow pressure

Your elbow is softened with an open arm angle and sharpened to a point when it is bent. It can be applied to heavily muscled areas, such as the hindquarters, the buttock in particular, and along the Bladder Meridian (if it is physically feasible and comfortable for you). When softened, it "tonifies"; bent to a point, it sedates. It can replace your tired thumb or fingertips. It is obviously less sensitive to energy than your hands, but can be developed as a sensitive tool. It is most useful for deeper penetration into tight, not pained, muscles, and for stronger specific pressure than you might easily give with your thumb or fingers. It should not be used in very sensitive, reactive areas.

An area should be warmed first with palm and perhaps fingertip pressure before using your elbow. You then apply the elbow as the moving pressure, while your supporting hand presses firmly, at first several

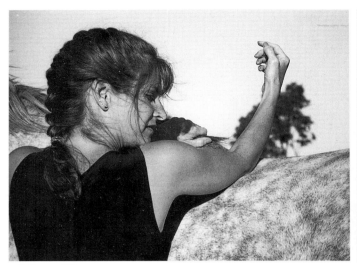 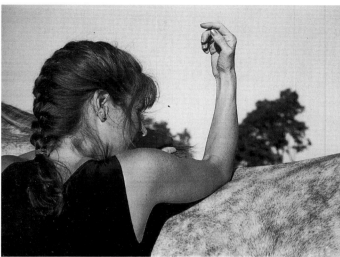

9.3a–c Elbow pressure.
9.3a *Pamela's arm is slightly bent to create a "soft" elbow, which she has placed on the Bladder Meridian. Her supporting hand is inches away. She is gradually dropping weight into her elbow and hand. This is a soft but specific pressure.*

9.3b *She is deepening the pressure by bending her forearm toward her shoulder.*

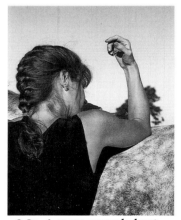

9.3c *A more severely bent arm and pointed elbow gives even deeper and more specific pressure, as the supporting hand presses firmly. Pamela is leaning her weight in from her center, not from her shoulder, and her hand and forearm are relaxed.*

inches away, to distract and comfort your horse. Never use your other elbow as the supporting pressure.

Gently place your open elbow on an area, and rest it there for a few seconds before pressing in. Fold your arm toward you to sharpen the angle of your elbow, as you lean your body weight into it and into your supporting hand, deepening the pressure. Hold. Slowly soften and release the pressure as you reopen the angle of your elbow/arm. (See Photos 9.3a–c.)

Use an open, soft elbow along the Bladder Meridian before you follow with the above technique, which applies deeper pressure.

Always keep your wrist, hand and fingers relaxed. Any tension in the hand will be felt as tension in the elbow, and you'll tire more easily.

Arm pressure
The back of your forearm, from the elbow to the wrist, may be used to work large areas. It can be used along a meridian, to bring warmth, for "tonification", or across muscles (not aligned with the fibers), to loosen and activate large areas, to "move" the muscle fibers. It is useful on the muscles of the shoulders, back and hindquarters.

Because your arm is a less sensitive sensing device, you should work the area first with your palms and/or fingertips to assess the condition of the muscles (tense? tight? painful?) and the energy flow, and how to proceed.

You may accompany arm pressure with a supporting hand, or use both arms simultaneously: one supports while the other actively "moves" energy. Your arms can alternate roles as they "step" across a muscle.

With your supporting hand or arm in place, you lean your weight into your forearm. Standing slightly away from your horse will allow you to lean in from your center. Your palm faces up, you use the back of the forearm. Your hand and wrist are relaxed. A tense hand creates a hard and tense arm, while a relaxed hand allows a comforting pressure. Arm pressure is more "tonifying", and should feel very comfortable to you both. It may even seem appropriate to gently lean your body against your horse's as you work. You should both relax and enjoy the contact. (See Photo 9.4.)

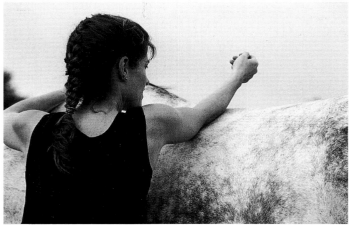

9.4 Arm pressure. Standing slightly away from Kate so she can lean in from her center, Pamela has laid the back of her forearm across Kate's back muscles to give "tonifying" pressure. A supporting hand rests on the withers.

Rotation and Stretching

The individual rotations and stretches are explained and illustrated in the Shiatsu treatment section, in the chapters dealing with the neck, the shoulders and forelegs, the hindquarters, and the tail and spine. Here we'll discuss their benefits and the general rules that apply to them.

We rotate the horse's forelegs (shoulders), hindlegs (hip joints), hooves (fetlocks), and tail vertebrae, and we stretch her legs, neck and tail (spine):

○ to improve circulation to the muscles and joints;
○ to activate the energy in all of the meridians passing through the joints;
○ to raise deeper meridians toward the skin for greater effectiveness with less pressure;
○ to release blocked energy in jitsu areas;
○ to release tightened muscle fibers;
○ to increase muscle tone, flexibility and range of motion;

○ to provide passive exercise during periods of recuperative confinement;
○ to give the horse awareness of and confidence in her extended physical abilities and possibilities;
○ to revitalize and create a sense of well-being.

Healing is promoted on a deeper level by rotations and stretches, because they activate the energy in the local meridians (six major meridians pass through each leg: three on the outside, and three on the inside). The major meridians at the surface interconnect with the lesser and deeper ones, and will reach the deeper muscles and tissue. They also reach their corresponding branches on the opposite side of the body, enabling you to work the meridians, muscles and joints of a non-injured side in order to promote the healing of a painful, unworkable injury on the opposite one.

Using pressure on a meridian or muscle in its stretched position, with the meridians raised and the muscles released from a tight, contracted condition, allows deeper and more effective healing. (See Photo 9.5.)

Rotations and stretches clarify the range of motion, and should be done just to the point of resistance, never forced. Rotations of the fore or hind legs should at first be small, then increased; as you enlarge their circumference, decrease their speed. There are times when a small rotation and stretch are more beneficial then extending to the full range of motion, which would aggravate damaged tissue rather than promote healing. The direction of your rotations, clockwise or counter-clockwise, will depend upon which muscles of your horse are to be affected: observe your horse's movement and your intuitive response. It is generally best, for flexibility and balance, to rotate in both directions, but specific problems create specific needs. You should complete your leg rotations with a crescendo-like stretch, a slight release, a slightly further stretch, then a slow release. You might repeat the process two or three times.

A stretch is done slowly and steadily and released slowly and steadily, with no sudden thrusts. The stretch is normally taken like a crescendo to what feels like the maximum, released a bit, then, if your horse permits, taken an inch or two further before a full release.

The techniques should be applied on both sides of your horse, unless an injury or painful resistance directs otherwise. Change sides frequently when working the legs, or your horse might remind you to do so.

We rotate the legs to give passive exercise to an injured limb or horse, and to promote freer and greater movement. We rotate the forelegs to rotate the shoulder muscles and joints and to reach the deeper muscles of the shoulder. Rotating the hind legs works upon the back muscles, the hip joints, the large and deep muscles of the hindquarters, and the joints, ligaments, tendons and muscles of the legs; it can relieve sore and tense muscle pain, and release muscle tightening around vertebrae and joints. Rotation and stretching of the hooves relieves tightening and soreness, increases circulation and mobility, and activates the flow of energy in the meridians. Rotation of the fetlock joint of the foreleg and of the tail vertebrae, bone by bone, helps to release tension in the upper neck.

Lateral stretches of the horse's neck serve to relieve tightened muscles and displaced vertebrae, to increase flexibility and mobility, and to relieve jaw tension and headaches. If your horse is resisting being "on the bit" or lateral flexion, the lateral neck stretches may relieve that resistance and develop suppleness in the muscles. They will also bring a (re)new(ed) awareness to a horse who travels stiffly on her forehand. As mentioned, rotations of the fetlock joint of the foreleg and of the tail vertebrae work to release tension in the upper neck. By the same laws of physiology of the spinal column and the nervous system, stretching and working the neck can relieve soreness and pain in the horse's lower back (loin), hindquarters (sacrum) and tail.

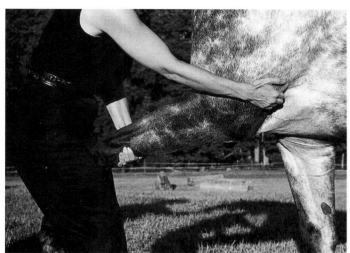

9.5 Fingertip pressure on the stretched and released muscle allows deeper and more effective healing.

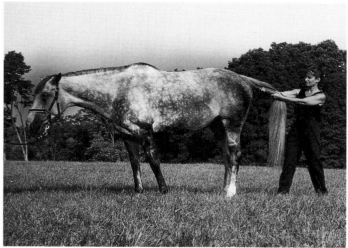

9.6 Full stretch of the tail and spine. Kate responds to the backward pull of her tail bone by straightening and lengthening her neck and leaning away, creating a full stretch of her spine from the last tail vertebra through her poll and down through her jaw.

Stretching the tail stretches the entire spine of the horse. It increases awareness and flexibility in the tail and in the entire spine, and it creates an energy flow that travels, through the vertebrae, nerves and Governing Vessel, directly to the head. It's a technique that horses enjoy; it feels good. The last vertebra of the tail relates directly to the first vertebra of the neck, and so on, and you therefore relieve problems in the neck by stretching and by rotating the vertebrae of the tail. Developing suppleness in the tail develops it through the body, and particularly in the neck. An uneven tail carriage may be corrected by these techniques, if the cause is tightened muscles. A horse who is not comfortable being touched around her tail and hind end will soon accept and even enjoy the tail exercises. Your veterinarian may be happily surprised by your horse's ease on her next rectal palpation. A tail and spine stretch (Photo 9.6) is a good way to end a session, for it imparts a sense of wholeness.

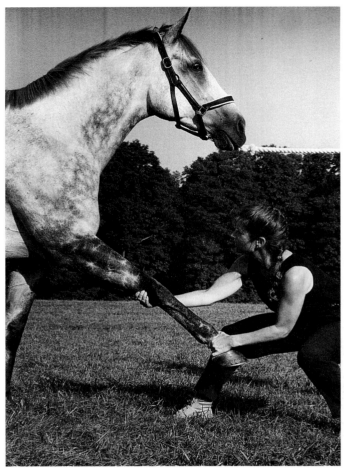

9.7 Move your entire body as a fluid unit. Support and move from your center, with your stance wide, knees bent, and weight on the balls of your feet. Your support should evoke your horse's confidence.

To move your horse's energy with these techniques, move your entire body as a fluid unit while you work (Photo 9.7). Particularly relax your shoulders, arms and hands. You support and move from your center, with your stance wide, your knees bent, and your weight on the balls of your feet. Your hold or pressure on the limb, whether it's a leg, the neck or the tail, should always evoke your horse's confidence in your supportive role. You fully support the leg from the moment you lift it off the ground to move it, to when you replace it on the ground, toe first, slowly and gently. You lift with lower-body strength, from your center.

If your horse's neck, leg or tail feels tense, send her the message to "relax" by focusing on your own relaxed energy and allowing her to feel it; feel her limb soften into your supportive hands.

Once horses learn a new range of motion and flexibility, with new sensations and awareness, they are, barring injury or continued aggravation, able to recreate and maintain it. It's similar to a rider learning the feeling of a horse moving in self-carriage, then recreating the motion by duplicating the feeling. For a horse this may entail self-rotation and stretch of a leg and/or, perhaps, shaking up energy with some creative leaps and bucks (see Photo 9.8) or a good roll.

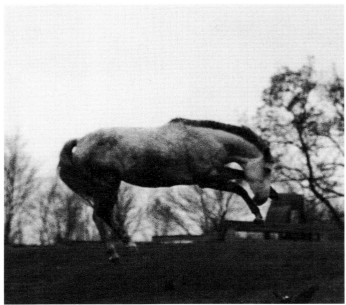

9.8 Self shiatsu. Kate uses a creative buck to stretch her spine from poll to dock and her forelegs forward.

"Jiggling"

A "jiggle" is Pamela's name for a to-and-fro and up-and-down flowing, rhythmic movement, done at a slow to medium tempo, softly, gently, never with a rough feel or jerking motion.

Its purpose is to move the energy within the joints and muscles, to loosen muscle fibers and relax the muscles, and to possibly send energy to or release energy from the deeper muscles. It is also used, simultaneously, to evaluate the range of muscle movement, at the beginning, during, and end of treatment.

The neck

You jiggle your horse's neck by placing both hands over the crest and moving it rhythmically toward and away from you. Move your hands as a unit and jiggle the length of the neck. You can move down and up its length, or up and down, and repeat as you need to. If the poll is sensitive, work beyond it and begin near the withers. If your horse's neck is

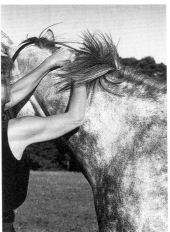
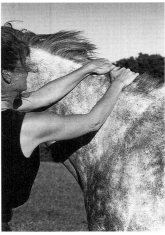
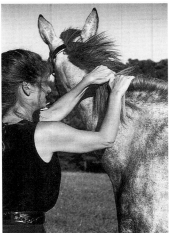

9.9a–c Jiggling the neck.
9.9a With her hands draped over the crest. Pamela's fingers press to gently move Katydid's neck towards her, as her elbows bend. She doesn't force movement, but stays sensitive to the degrees of possibility.

9.9b Now the heels of her palms push Kate's neck away, with help from her upper and lower arms as her elbows straighten.

9.9c She rhythmically continues this to and fro movement, as her hands progressively slide down the crest toward the withers. Here you can see how the neck has softened, bending easily with the motion.

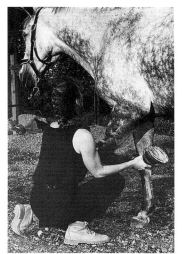

9.10 Jiggling the shoulder. With the lower leg supported parallel to the ground, gently push and pull the knee away and toward you, rhythmically, as though you were swinging the knee from side to side. Observe the degree of movement rippling through the muscles and joints of the upper leg and shoulder.

tense, sensitive or resistant, the jiggle should relax it, loosen its energy, and prepare it for pressure and stretching. (See Photos 9.9a–c.)

The shoulders

The jiggle is an important technique for the evaluation and treatment of the shoulder musculature.

○ Pick up your horse's leg, kneel down, and rest it on your knee. She must feel assured, by a confident and comfortable posture, that your knee is there to support her. (See Photo 9.10.)

○ Keep the lower leg parallel to the ground.

○ With one hand supporting her fetlock and foot, place your other hand on her knee to move it up and down and toward and away from you, as though you were swinging the knee from side to side. It's a loosening movement that flows back and forth to move and release the muscles and joints above, through the forearm, elbow, upper arm and shoulder. You are relaxing the muscles and beginning to move the energy in and around them.

○ Observe the movement, the degree and extent of the rippling waves, and the resiliency of the muscles.

○ Gently replace the foot on the ground, and change sides.

Once you are rotating and stretching the leg and shoulder complex, you may use the jiggle to further release the muscles and joints and to confirm their loosening as you progress.

○ Stand facing your horse's chest, just to the outside of the leg you will lift.
○ Place one hand over the other, behind and just above her knee.
○ Raise her forearm as close to parallel with the ground as is comfortable for her, without force or strain.
○ Your hold must be supportive. (See Photo 9.11.)
○ Softly swing the leg from side to side and up and down, while you watch the shoulder muscles move and the elbow flex.

You can repeat this movement throughout the rotation and stretching treatment, and at its end. It will serve as a final loosening and release. Note any changes in the nature and degree of motion.

The standing-leg jiggle is done with the leg weighted on the ground. You use it when you first begin the shoulder and foreleg treatment and at its end, for evaluating and releasing the muscles. It can also be used intermittently during treatment, when you are changing sides. It is very useful if your horse is uncomfortable having you lift and support her leg.
○ Kneel beside your horse's leg.
○ Place a hand on either side of her forearm, a few inches above the knee.
○ Use gentle but firm palm pressure to slightly, softly, pull the leg toward you and release in a repetitive, rhythmic motion, so the shoulder muscles "bounce" with your movement.
○ Observe the muscles.

The hindquarters

Jiggling the hindquarters through the leg allows you to evaluate the general tightness and tone of the muscles of the entire area, as well as relax the muscles and release blocked energy.
○ When your horse places her hind leg in the resting position (or you ask her to do so by lifting and placing it yourself), with the foot tilted off the ground and rested on its toe, the large muscles of the leg and hindquarters are released into a relaxed state. We jiggle the leg when it's in this released position.
○ With your supporting hand over the front of the gaskin, or resting just above the fetlock, your moving hand gently rocks the hock from side to side. (See Photo 9.12.) The leg will seem to swing loosely, pivoting on the toe.
○ Try, in this way, to observe all the visible muscles in the hindquarters moving. You should be able to see the muscles move about the hip socket.

Use this technique to evaluate or confirm the condition of the muscles in the area, use it when you begin work on the hindquarters, and use it again to confirm the loosening effects of the hind-leg rotations.

As you use the technique of jiggling, mentally visualize the total relaxation of the muscles, the muscle fibers, and the release of blocked energy within.

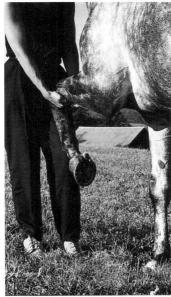

9.11 One hand over the other, behind and just above the knee, comfortably raises Kate's forearm parallel to the ground. The upper leg is softly swung side to side and up and down, as Pamela watches the shoulder muscles and elbow move.

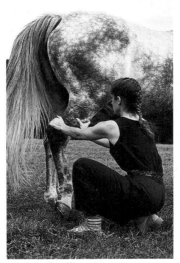

9.12 Jiggling the hindquarters. With the leg in the released rest position, the hock is gently rocked from side to side. This loosens the muscles, releases blocked energy, and allows diagnosis of muscle condition.

Percussion

Percussion is used on muscles:
○ to release blocked energy;
○ to wake up the nervous system;
○ to increase circulation to an area;
○ to release muscle tension;
○ to bring awareness to the horse of where she needs to release;
○ to enliven a very relaxed horse at the end of a session;
○ to sedate an overly energized horse.

It is not used on injured or sore muscles, swollen tissue, nor sensitive areas.

Your hands are cupped loosely together to form a pocket of air between your palms. Your forearms and hands move as a unit hinged at your elbows, but your wrists are loose and flexible. You hold your cupped hands 2–4 inches from your horse's body and release your arms and wrists to make contact with the back of one hand. The contact should be vertical, at ninety degrees to the body surface. You should hear a whooshing sound as the pocket of air absorbs the impact. Your cupped hands should "bounce" back up from contact, not pound into the body. The muscles should undulate in response to your contacts. (See Photos 9.13 a–d.)

The movement is repeated quickly and rhythmically along and across muscled areas, at intervals of 1 inch to 3–4 inches. The distance of the intervals, the distance between on-and-off body contact, and the degree of pressure on contact (light to heavy) will depend upon:

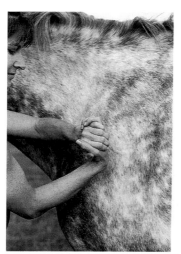 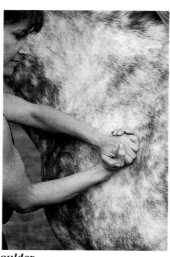 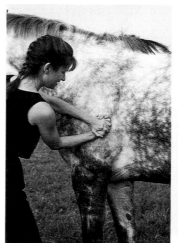 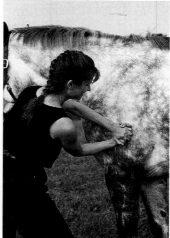

9.13a–d Percussion on the shoulder.
9.13a Hold your cupped hands two to three inches from the muscle and ...

9.13b ... release your arms and wrists to percuss the muscle. There should be a whooshing sound as the pocket of air between your palms absorbs the impact.

9.13c Move down an inch and "hit" again.

9.13d Another inch and "hit" again. These three taps took one second. Pamela is working a circular pattern over the groups of muscles, and avoiding bone.

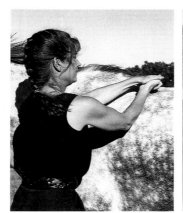 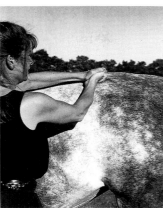 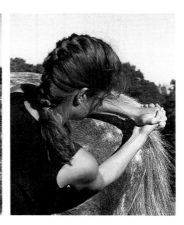

9.14a–b Percussion along the back.

9.14a From two to three inches away, the back of the hand makes light contact along the Bladder Meridian and the large longissimus dorsi muscle, then "bounces" up, …

9.14b … keeping a steady one two rhythm as it follows the meridian and the muscle. The wrists stay flexible and relaxed.

9.15 On the hindquarters, percussions originate from three to four inches off the body, and occur at intervals of three to four inches. Contacts are firm and rhythmic. You should be able to see the muscles undulate with contact.

- the depth of the muscle mass;
- the size of the area you are working;
- the tightness of the muscles;
- whether you want to calm the horse or to enliven her.

You repeat two to three times your entire pattern of movements, which are either circular over a large muscled area, or linear following the muscle fibers or a meridian.

If your horse is reactive to this technique, shows sensitivity, or seems to not enjoy it, don't pursue it in that area. You may try to continue it elsewhere, where her muscles will relax from the activity. Percussion stimulates, to rebalance the body's energy: applied properly, it will calm or enliven and stimulate muscles to relax, though it may at first sound contradictory. It should not be used on an overly stimulated (sensitive, painful, inflamed) area; in such a case, jiggling, which is slow and gentle, may be used instead.

On the **shoulders**, use small, close movements with 1-inch intervals and not much distance between on-and-off contact. Two "hits" will take one second or less. You can work in a circular pattern or follow the length of the muscle fibers of the various groups. Repeat several times.

Use the same small, close movements along the **back** (Photos 9.14 a–b). Keep your contact quick and light. Follow the length of the large longissimus dorsi muscle from the withers to the sacrum. Percussion is very effective along the Bladder Meridian, and you can follow it through to the buttock and down the hamstring muscles. Take care to stay off bones. This technique would be used on the back after using pressure, not before, and not if any soreness remains.

Larger, stronger movements and heavier contact are used on the deeper and larger muscles of the **hindquarters** (Photo 9.15). Contact originates from farther off the body, and occurs at intervals of 3—4 inches. Here, too, you can work in a circular pattern or follow the length of the muscles. Remember to repeat the pattern two to three times.

Percussion may be used on the **neck** after using pressure and stretching techniques. Use gentle contact, with small, close movements at 1-inch intervals, and follow the muscles, vertebrae and meridian lines. (See Photos 9.16a—c.) Begin approximately 5 inches below the poll, with

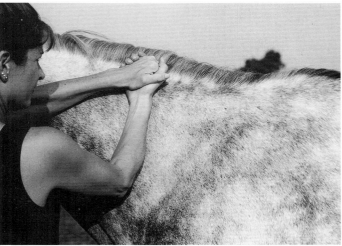

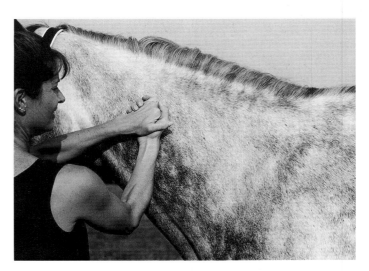

9.16a—c Percussion on the neck.
*9.16a Follow the Bladder Meridian from **beyond** the sensitive poll to the withers. Begin with very light, gentle taps and increase their intensity as you move onto heavier muscle. Repeat this line one or two times.*

9.16b Now percuss down the lateral midline of the neck, over the cervical vertebrae. Use gentle, small taps until the muscles deepen before and over the shoulder blade. Repeat.

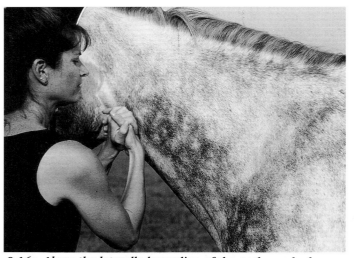

9.16c Along the laterally lower line of the neck, work above the line of the jugular groove. The Large Intestine Meridian runs here. Push the back of your cupped hands upward, to percuss at a 90° angle, using small, close, gentle movements until you reach the lower shoulder. Repeat.

very light taps. "Hit" a little harder with each tap as you move down toward and onto the shoulder, following out the muscle. On the neck of a horse who carries tension in her jaw, poll and/or neck, percussion, even applied gently, will be too jarring; the jiggling technique would serve well.

To calm a nervous or highly energized horse, use firmer pressure, larger and faster movements, and cover more body area in less time.

You enliven a quiet horse with light, quick pressure from small, close movements. This will stimulate and make her aware of her own body. Use this technique at the end of a session preceding a show, or to awaken your sleepy horse before a class.

To use percussion on a quiet horse whom you want to remain quiet, keep your hands close to her body and use smoother, less stacatto movements.

Percussion is often used near the end of a session, following other techniques. Follow percussion with stroking (see TECHNIQUES: Stroking, p. 76) to quiet your horse's energy. You will leave her feeling relaxed, yet alert and aware of the changes going on within.

Moving Muscle

This technique is used mainly on the large muscles of the hindquarters, on the gluteus maximus and the biceps femoris muscles. A modified version can be used on the neck, shoulders and back. It improves circulation and flexibility. It's an important technique to use on an area sensitive to touch, for it should be less painful than direct, vertical pressure.

A supporting arm is draped across your horse's spine, and your supporting hand gives firm but gently opposing pressure. A relaxed, moving hand lays across the muscle and molds to it. You lean weight obliquely

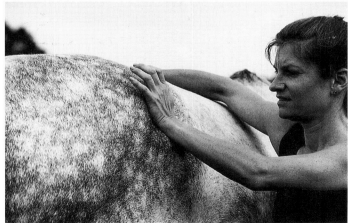
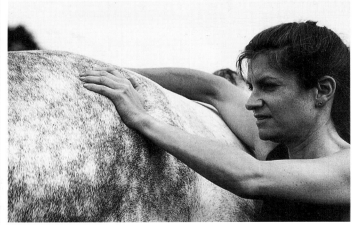

9.17a–b Moving muscle.
9.17a Leaning into the heel of the moving hand causes the muscle to bulge upward and fill the palm.

9.17b The fingers then press down and in to slightly pull the muscle down. A supporting arm and hand firmly hold against the pressure on the other side of the spine.

(rather than vertically) into the heel of your palm, feel the muscle rise up and fill your hand, lean in more pressure so the muscle bulges further upward, then press in and down with your fingertips, to pull the muscle slightly down. Repeat this two or three times. Then move your hand rearward over the muscle about 2 inches and repeat. You'll be able to repeat this technique two to four times across the muscle. (See Photos 9.17a–b.)

You can also "move muscle" with your forearm or with the cupped-hands position that you use for percussion. You lay the back of your forearm or the back of one of your cupped hands against the muscle and, without removing contact, rhythmically press, release, press, release, press, release, and so on, retaining contact on release. The angle of your pressure should be softly oblique rather than vertical and direct. You will see a ripple effect in the surrounding area. Your cupped hands may be used on shoulder, back and hindquarter muscles, your forearm on the neck (supported), shoulders, back and hindquarters.

10 *Treating Kyo and Jitsu, Imbalances within YinYang*

Yin and Yang are the two aspects of one thing, the inseparable duality that, in the Oriental view, characterizes the nature of everything. The Yin aspect is interior, hidden, quiet, subtle, more delicate, and receptive; the Yang is outgoing, energized, warm and bright like the sun. Everything that exists has more or less of one and the other, and the balance is in constant flux. Because one aspect generally dominates, a being or a thing is said to be either Yin or Yang or, more accurately, **Yin**Yang or Yin**Yang**. There are Yin-type people and Yang-type people, though both generalized types possess qualities and behavioral characteristics of the other in variable degrees. This, naturally, applies to horses as well.

A generalized Yin-type horse may have more refined physical features, be reticent, perhaps timid, and be more sensitive emotionally and physically. This type may be more markedly disturbed by changes in routine or environment, be a fussy eater or difficult "keeper", develop symptoms of illness or injury more gradually over a longer period, and take longer to recover.

A Yang-type horse may look physically more powerful, with more bone and muscle, perhaps have less-refined features, and be confident mentally and physically, competitive, aggressive, and dominant. This type is highly energized, and may "burn out" before the course is run. A Yang type is more injury-prone, but recovers quickly.

A particular dis-ease or disease in an individual is characterized as well by the quality of either Yin or Yang, as are points on the meridians and areas on the body. Kyo and jitsu are the two conditions of a YinYang imbalance of energy that is dis-ease and eventually disease. Kyo is the lack and need of Ki energy, while jitsu is an over-accumulation of it. If a point or an area is excessively Yin, it is kyo; if it's excessively Yang, it's jitsu. If the condition or disease has exhausted the animal, or person, it's a kyo condition; if an excess of energy has caused blockage and the resultant problems, it's a jitsu condition.

When a very Yin-type horse is ailing or an ailing horse has a kyo condition, her store of energy is low. Such a horse needs sensitive, gentle and supportive treatment. The shiatsu technique for this treatment is "tonification". It employs gentle, soothing pressure that is increased very gradually and held for an extended length of time, thirty to sixty seconds, then very slowly released. You "tonify" the weakest point on the meridian or part of the area: it may feel cool or cold, be visibly sinking in or hollow-looking, or just give that sensation and seem to pull in your touch; you will feel little if any movement of energy; it will feel silent and empty, or almost so. Hold, in most cases with palm pressure, until you feel a response, a pulsing, a tingling, a filling of the void, or just a sense that it's time to release. *Zen Shiatsu* tells us to wait as we hold, "... affectionately, patiently, and without regard to time", so the nurturing warmth can reach deep within to strengthen and normalize the area.

When you treat a kyo condition, except in cases of extreme depletion and fatigue, you may find areas of jitsu. Treat them with caution, using the stimulating techniques very conservatively. Take care not to further consume the energy, but rather to redirect it toward the prime area of kyo that is in need. Don't over-stretch, jiggle gently, smoothly and slowly, and percuss using small, close and smooth movements. Work slowly. The stimulation/sedation techniques of strong, deep, and quick pressure and vigorous movement should not be used. As happens when we over-exercise, over-stimulation could further deplete the horse's low energy and leave her exhausted, possibly dangerously so; the healing process could be prolonged rather than enhanced. It's also true that over-use of stimulation/sedation techniques can create a kyo condition, by exhausting the energy.

With a Yin-type horse, and with kyo conditions, you must be patient, for it may take longer to see a response to treatment and recovery. It's important to remember that when your horse, or her muscle or organ, has been stressed and exhausted, she is that much more susceptible to injury or re-injury. Tonification activates the healing process deep within to rebuild energy and strength. Your horse gradually will be able to accommodate more stimulating shiatsu and more strenuous activity, and her personality may change as her energy level, strength and self-confidence grow.

Excessive Yang-type horses and jitsu conditions are treated with stimulation/sedation techniques. Although it may sound like a contradiction, continuous stimulation is sedating. For the healing process to be fully activated, the horse, or a particular area of her body, must relax and release the over-accumulation of energy. To accomplish this, match the strength and speed of the techniques to the horse's energy and personality. Generally, stronger, more penetrating, sharper and quicker pressure is used, along with larger movements. The fingertips, thumbs and elbows apply pressure. Stretches are taken to their maximum, slightly released, then stretched again to just beyond. The other techniques of rotation, jiggling, percussion and "moving muscle" are also used. The jitsu areas are much easier to find, and to treat, than the kyo. It takes less effort and time to release energy than to replenish it. Jitsu may feel tight, hard, hot, rapidly pulsating, maybe vibrating. To fully treat a jitsu condition, you must seek out the principal kyo area or condition, which is the source of the problem, tonify it, and send it the released energy from the jitsu area.

11 *Quieting a Nervous Horse*

It's hard to do anything around an overly energized horse. Neither of you can focus on your task while her energy is diverted. It's especially frustrating when you're trying to help your horse, but she's a 1200 lb moving target and weapon. (I could give a book of testimony on this subject.) However, because I'm at least as stubborn as my mare, I've found techniques that work with her, most times, if I patiently persevere. Pamela, on the other hand, on a professional call, must divine a way to reach whatever horse personality is her client of the moment.

Pamela, firstly, exudes calmness and confidence at all times with the horse. She uses soothing talk, and laughter, because horses seem to respond so well to the sounds of both. Occasionally she uses soothing and unobtrusive meditation-type music. Before the session begins, she may do something to bring the horse's interest to herself, such as ignoring the horse into investigating her. Sometimes she takes the horse for a walk and a chat, "listing all the things I'm going to do and how we're going to have a wonderful time working together to help him. While we're walking I begin the work by touching here and there and watching his eyes so that I know what he'll respond to and enjoy if he gets distracted later. I may walk him every five minutes during the session, all the while keeping my attention on him and giving him a lot of different kinds of stimulation."

The session begins with the stroking technique. If it calms, it's used for a longer period of time. Sometimes she stops stroking before she loses the horse's attention, so the horse will ask for more, then strokes for a slightly longer period of time, then withdraws, and so on, until the horse relaxes and focuses on the session.

Mirroring the horse's high energy in her degree of pressure and the tempo and size of her movements has a sedating effect, particularly with the use of percussion and jiggling. Inviting the horse to mirror her calm, quiet confidence can also work its spell: she leans on the horse, shoulder to shoulder, so her deep, rhythmic breathing is felt and heard.

Pamela doesn't always have the advantage of time. There are sessions when she has to literally reach in with quick accuracy and accept that less help will do and be better than none. An extreme example was the case of a six-million-dollar syndicated stallion. His sperm count was down and his desire was lost.

> "He was resentful of any human contact, and was placed in cross-ties (chains, to be exact) by someone resembling the Incredible Hulk. He stomped, struck out, and generally tried to project a macho image. The Hulk stood by the horse's head

while I tentatively reached out and pressed the points I had read were used for impotence. This was not a heartwarming experience and left me frustrated. I realized I had to let go of my ego and expectations. A week or two later, I ran into the stallion's veterinarian. 'By the way,' he said, disbelievingly, 'your timing was immaculate. Not only did his sperm count go up drastically, but his desire has returned.' I asked that the next foal be named after me."

For your horse to benefit most fully from shiatsu, and from your efforts, she must relax, release tension, and direct her attention and energy toward the healing process that you are promoting within her.

12 *Touching Pain*

Sometimes your horse jumps from your touch. You've approached a sensitive spot, one either holding pain or associated with pain, physically or emotionally. Or you've approached an area unaccustomed to touch. You want to gradually introduce your touch and the use of therapeutic pressure to the area.

You begin by touching elsewhere. Work the adjacent areas if you can. If the pain or discomfort is in the:

○ **Neck** – treat the shoulder first.
○ **Shoulder** – work the neck and gently rotate and stretch the forelegs before attempting pressure on the shoulder.
○ **Leg** – use very slow and gentle leg jiggles and rotations and modified stretches to move the painful energy without pressure directly upon it; support the limb well through these manipulations so that the horse is not using her own muscles.
○ **Head, ear** or **poll** – begin with gently soothing but firm pressure at the base of the neck or within the zone where your horse feels safe and comfortable.
○ **Hind end** – especially if she kicks, it's important to desensitize this area; begin where she is comfortable and gradually work with firm, supportive pressure toward the tail, progressing as she allows and learns to welcome it.

Desensitization could take one session, weeks, or possibly months. Work trustingly and without regard to time.

When I got Katydid as a three-year-old, she didn't kick, but she didn't like her tail to be touched. So I made a point of often changing sides via close contact with her tail and a firm, brief hand-caress upon it. This merely became part of my routine, and still is. My touch there was soon accepted, then welcomed; this probably took months. Our veterinarian was surprised and relieved that she relaxed and readily accepted her first rectal palpation. I think that Katy's tail is now her favorite place for my caress, for she's learned to associate it with my care and with healing and well-being. When she's in pain, or simply tensely distracted, I can reach her through her tail.

> Spring injections that year caused three-out-of-three reactions, but Katy was by far the worst. She stood in her stall with her neck hung off her shoulder, but could not lower it a few more inches to her dinner. By morning, she stood propped up by her hind end pressed against the stall wall. Her entire body seemed in spasm. I spent most of the day with her, listening

to classical music from my tape recorder and unknotting her tail, hair by hair. By the end of the day, she accepted my touch on her hindquarters. The following day I was able to work along her Bladder Meridian, from the withers to the hocks. By evening I could touch the other side of her neck, the side without the painful swelling. The third morning, I palmed slowly along her Bladder Meridian, then on the neck's unswollen side. I moved to the painful side and began palm pressure along the outer limits, slowly, ever so slowly holding, then inching in toward the swelling. At last I was allowed to place a soft, warm hand on the inflamed injection site: Katy released a huge sigh and, with it, the tension that had held her body for four days. She walked out of her stall to rejoin her pasture-mates.

Sometimes there is too much pain. A traumatized area is overly stimulated by the bodily response and should not be touched. Pamela describes this as jitsu protecting and hiding the underlying kyo. Once the area will accept touch, it will need tonification, not sedation. Until that time, you may hold your hand closely over the area to radiate warmth to it. Your supporting hand strokes or scratches nearby, to soothe and distract. Hold at first for a few seconds, then increase the time, but still do not touch. Pamela suggests:

> "When touching without actually touching, imagine that you are sending healing energy to the pain, or imagine the pain rising out of your horse. Some people like to imagine white light going to the pain, or some other soothing color. Imagine that color coming out of the area."

Eventually, touch lightly as a feather, for a moment, then gradually longer. Then you may begin to combine touching the surrounding areas as well, as gently. You may increase your pressure as you sense it is needed and acceptable, always observing and responding to your horse's responses. You want to gain and hold your horse's trust.

To affect but not touch an overly sensitive area, you may, where you can, work along the meridian that runs through it and on its corresponding branch and specific area on the opposite side. The movement of energy informs and aids an impaired area through a corresponding one.

The stroking technique is one way to begin to touch a sensitive area (see TECHNIQUES: Stroking, p. 78). Use a light and gentle contact, stroking palm over palm over this part of the body. Move over the non-sensitive surrounding areas as well, then again over the sensitive one, and so forth.

Your use of palm pressure begins distally from the sensitive point, and slowly works towards it. Once your touch is accepted at the painful site, your pressure is gentle, with just the weight and warmth of your relaxed hand conforming to the contour of the body. Increase the pressure slowly but firmly, as it is tolerated. Your supporting hand should be close by, where there is no sensitivity. It's used to distract from and to help move the painful energy. If need be, it applies as much or more pressure than your moving hand, and it may squeeze, scratch or tap to distract.

If you allow your horse time to gain confidence in your touch and movements, she may knowingly welcome you to a zone of discomfort.

Chapter end note

While writing this chapter, I was a passenger in a near head-on collision. I had only the section on untouchable pain to finish, and so I wrote it as I experienced it and the process of healing.

Pamela postponed our scheduled work date from the second to the fourth day following the trauma, explaining that my pain would be untouchable until then. Although I was in pain, her touch was never painful. At a point during the session, a sense of well-being swelled and flowed through me; it stayed with me. By the session's end, I felt no longer depleted but, in fact, quite energized and noticeably better. The effect was lasting.

I observed my injuries and new incapacitations. I felt the value of being very conscious, even with a concussion, of my body, its sensations, its limitations, when I could begin to stretch my neck and back and to what degree, how to move, when to move and when to rest. I observed myself as I try to observe my horse, not in the future or past, not with expectations or regrets. I didn't dwell on nor in my pain and problems; I oberved them as I experienced them and responded to them, moment to moment. I was able to guide and enhance the healing of my bodymind, through my own watchfulness and through Pamela's gift of a shiatsu session.

I took no pain killers and no medications other than arnica, the homeopathic* remedy for shock, trauma, bruises, muscular injury and general healing. Pain killers would have silenced my body; I needed to hear it speak, or risk re-injuring torn and weakened tissue.

* Homeopathy is a medical system of remedies that treats the patient as an entire energetic system. It is explained in Appendix B.

13 *Keeping Your Horse Whole*

Stroking

- "Stroking" activates your horse's energy, wakes up her nervous system on a superficial and possibly deeper level.
- It gently introduces your touch to her entire body.
- It stimulates within her a physical sensation of wholeness, an awareness of where she begins and ends.
- It becomes the beginning sign of an enjoyable ritual you share together.

You use very relaxed, softly and slightly cupped hands, your fingers touching each other or slightly apart (not squeezed together). Your relaxed hands mold to the contours of your horse's body as they lightly glide over it. A light touch is essential. You make long, smooth, sweeping strokes in a hand-over-hand rhythmic motion that is similar to swimming the crawl, moving your entire arm from the shoulder socket. Your tempo may be slow or swift (match your horse's energy). Stroking is done in less than a minute.

Begin at the top of her neck and work toward the tail, going over the withers and down the shoulder and foreleg, across the back, sides and hindquarters, and down the hindlimb. Then repeat on the other side of her body, keeping physical contact as you change sides. (See Photos 13.1a–p.)

Finishing your session with stroking, after having worked on various areas of her body, will renew for your horse the sensation of being whole, rather than a collection of parts.

Maintaining Physical Contact

There are times when you will be moving back and forth every few minutes to work on one side of your horse's body and then the other. This will occur when you're doing leg rotations and stretches, when you're using percussion and stroking techniques, when you want to immediately compare from side to side the effect of your work, when your horse becomes too relaxed on the side where you're working and therefore too uncomfortable on the unworked side, and when your horse has a short attention span. By maintaining physical contact with your horse as you move from side to side, you will establish a sense of continuum for your horse, yourself and your shiatsu session. You'll maintain a sense of wholeness and avoid the sense that you're working body parts. If your horse becomes so relaxed that she dozes, your continuous contact will prevent her from being startled. Maintaining contact helps to maintain trust between you.

Taking Breaks

A break allows your horse time to relax and feel, and to think about the changes and new sensations within her. It's time for her to move her own energy and make adjustments. It's time for you to observe how she is reacting and moving, to reassess the progress of the session. And it's time for you to rest and recenter your own energy.

A break can be taking your horse for a short, relaxed walk, turning her out alone or in a roomy stall for a few minutes, or giving a moment to encouraging words, a relaxed breath and refocusing yourself. It can also be encouraging your horse to move (stay relaxed, don't force), at whatever gait is appropriate for your assessment of her progress, with the assistance of a helper or lunge line if necessary.

Giving your horse some quiet time alone is imperative at the end of your session. She should be allowed to wander and experience what is happening in her body, and make still further adjustments.

Often, horses roll when turned out during a break or after treatment, and this is a wonderful way to self-adjust, rebalance and feel whole. Some horses strut and show off their renewed sense of well-being. Some do dynamic gallops, leaps and turns. Others thoughtfully, quietly stand, stroll or graze.

A thoroughbred gelding, who was distraught, aggressive and lame after being moved from the only home he had known, became calm and sound during Pamela's treatment. At the session's end, he took himself for a methodical and rhythmic ten-minute walk around the perimeter of the arena, in his difficult direction. He seemed to be in deep concentration, as he felt the renewed fluidity in his stride and sense of wholeness and calm. He thereafter accepted his new home and, in fact, quickly became the darling of the barn.

It's not uncommon for a horse to not immediately realize that a disability has gone, and to take the first few steps after treatment showing the same problem you have just worked to eliminate; within moments, the horse realizes that she no longer has to move in that distorted manner, and will then move correctly. Pamela has many stories to illustrate this.

> "When I finished the treatment session, this horse, who had been very lame, was turned out alone in the indoor arena. He started to walk with the same limp he had had; then his face changed: he realized that the pain was no longer there, nor the need to move in that incorrect manner. He took off in a gallop across the arena, stopped short before a mirror, looked at himself, then galloped on to his owner to bestow thankful kisses upon her.
>
> "In another incident, which occurred during an Essex three-day event, I was called to try to help a horse who had 'tied-

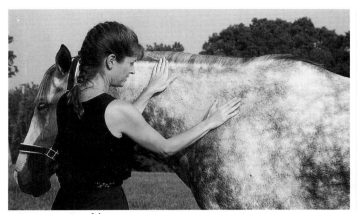

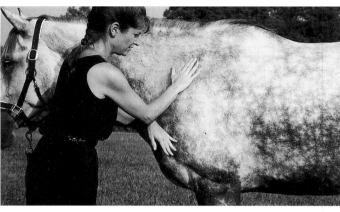

13.1a–p *Stroking.*
13.1a *Pamela began with her right hand at the top of Katy's neck, behind the poll: as it slides across to the shoulder, her left hand is placed midway on the neck to begin its stroke.*

13.1b *Her left hand now glides to the shoulder and down the front of the blade with one large sweeping motion. Her right hand, sustaining continuous movement, has been lifted off the body and repositioned on the shoulder.*

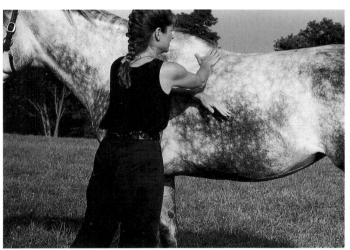

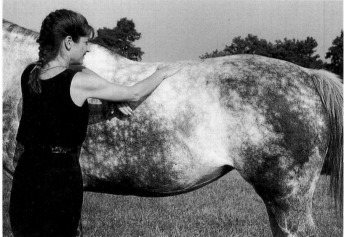

13.1f *Her right arm crosses back to begin a new stroke as her left hand ends one.*

13.1g *She progresses, hand over hand, across and over Kate's body.*

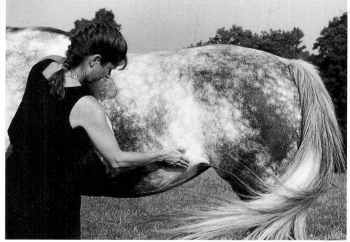

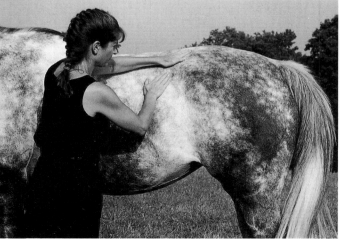

13.1j *... and across; ...*

13.1k *... the left reaches up to stroke over the loin; the right prepares ...*

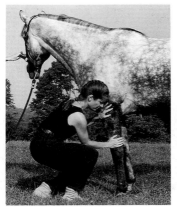

13.1c *Her left hand continues on to Kate's leg, and the right hand follows in another stroke, molding to the contour of the body.*

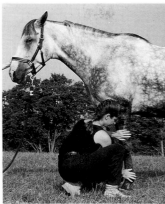

13.1d *With two more strokes, the right hand sweeps down to Kate's ankle and pastern. The left hand follows.*

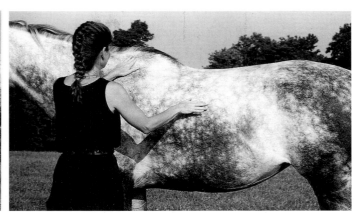

13.1e *Pamela rises, maintaining contact and rhythm. Her right hand sweeps across the shoulder and rib cage, and her left hand begins to follow.*

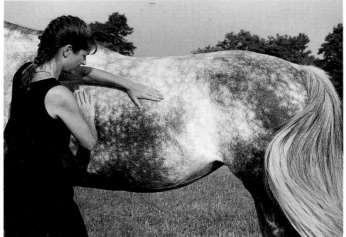

13.1h *Her left arm finishes a stroke across and down; her right hand prepares to begin. The hands follow the hair.*

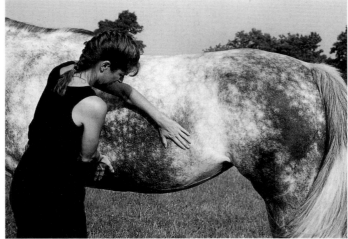

13.1i *The left hand glides across; the right hand crosses under . . .*

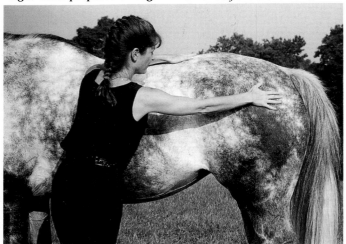

13.1l *. . . to pass over the pelvis to the hip; and the left hand prepares . . .*

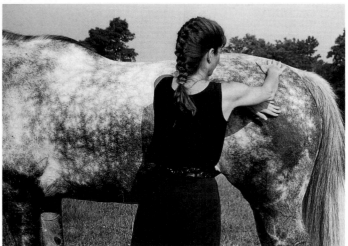

13.1m *. . . to glide over and down. The right crosses over to next stroke down the buttock.*

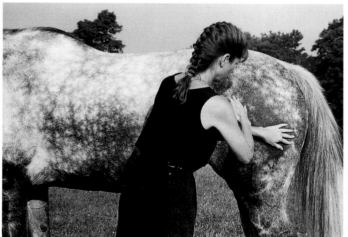

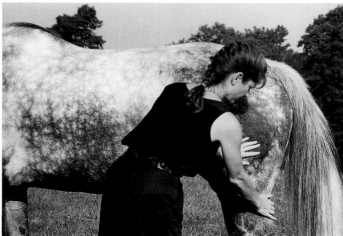

13.1n The left hand sweeps down, conforming to the muscle beneath it that it softly but quickly caresses. The right crosses over for the next stroke . . .

13.1o . . . *toward the hock. The left hand begins to follow.*

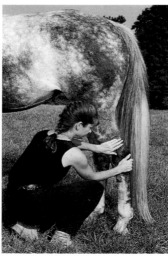

13.1p The left hand ends its stroke at the hock, as the right hand prepares to sweep down the lower leg. Pamela has followed the movement down with a centered and comfortably positioned body: her weight is balanced on the balls of her feet, with the wide enough stance of one leg in front of the other; she is able to stand up or move out of the way effortlessly and instantly. With at least one hand in contact with Kate's body, Pamela will now move to repeat on the other side.

up', and who had a history of this problem. I was told that in the past, in spite of the administered drugs, he had not been able to walk for twenty-four hours following an episode. After fifteen minutes of applying shiatsu pressure technique, I moved away to allow him to move. He stood for a moment, believing that, as in the past, he could not. Then he took a tentative step, and walked easily out of his stall and onto the lawn to graze. His amazed owner followed the tug of the lead rope wearing a huge grin."

Pamela warns:

"Sometimes there is a delayed response to the session. It may take a day for improvement to really show as the body continues to heal. The nature of some injuries will require rest and gradual reintroduction to work for the muscles to redevelop to support the body in the balanced position."

Rolling

Have you noticed how satisfied and relaxed a horse looks after a roll, or does your dismay over the "pigpen look" cloud your view? Katydid springs to her feet, her sleek silvery form smeared with thick brown mud, her cheeks rouged with our local red clay; she seems to wear a huge grin, punctuated with extraordinary aerial feats. I wonder at her moves, groan at the mess, and smile at her healthy gestures. Rolling is for horses one of the important means to self-heal and maintain health. It can dislodge and rebalance blocked energy, release tight muscles, realign vertebrae, stimulate circulation and the nervous system, relieve itchy spots, loosen dirt and dead hair and skin, absorb sweat with newly applied dirt, and let a horse feel whole rather than a collection of parts.

During Katydid's first treatment session with Pamela, she rolled during one or two of the many breaks. I gasped, probably because that's what every horse owner I had known did when their well-groomed horses rolled. Pamela assured me that it was the best thing that she could do for herself.

"I love to watch the horses I've worked on go out and wander around after a session. I enjoy seeing them rediscover their bodies and sometimes even look a bit uncertain about what's happened to them. Sometimes they express their feelings of peacefulness by grazing comfortably or exploring the area. Sometimes they leap and tear around because the energy that's just been released must have an outlet. But when they roll, I feel that it's like their corrective exercises. They adjust themselves in a way I couldn't possibly do, but because I've loosened them up, stretched them out, and relaxed them, they are now able to stretch more, perhaps roll on a vertebra that has been sticking up too high and push it back into place, or manipulate the vertebrae adjacent to one that has slipped downward so that it may be released up into the proper alignment. If a horse rolls and then takes a nap, it's even better. This gives the body a chance to use its energy for healing, rather than for moving, digesting or otherwise."

SECTION III

SHIATSU TREATMENT

14   *Treatment Guidelines*

A List of Reminders and Hints

○ **LISTEN to your horse** with your eyes, your hands, your body, and your inner ear.

○ **TALK in a soft, relaxed voice** to relax and reassure your horse. Low humming or singing, laughter, and words of reassurance and admiration can give you your horse's attention, give her confidence, and defuse tension.

○ **Work in a quiet ENVIRONMENT** where both your horse and you feel relaxed and safe.

○ **BREATHE deeply, rhythmically**. Allow your diaphragm to descend and your abdomen, lower back, sides, ribs and chest to expand, as your elastic lungs fill with air from the bottom up.

   Be aware of your horse's breathing patterns. Mirroring them may help you to understand her.

○ **STAND balanced, centered, with knees flexed**, with a wide stance to give yourself a stable base. Your weight should be on the balls of your feet, ready to instantly respond (do not sit back on your heels). Your movement and strength come from your center, in your lower torso. Your knees stay springy, never locked. You lower by bending your knees, not your waist, and lift from your center in your pelvis, with lower-body strength and your knees bent.

○ **MOVE your energy** to move your horse's. You are better able to feel her range of motion, affect it, support it, and know its limits when you move your whole body with hers, in concert with her energy.

   Match the speed of your movements to her energy. If she seems anxious or unsettled, gradually slow your speed and visualize her slowed, quiet, relaxed: her energy may now follow yours to a calmer state. Be aware that nervous horses often make humans nervous, and nervous humans create nervous horses: it's an example of one matching the energy of the other, but one that you don't want to follow. If you feel this happening, recenter yourself, visualize yourself calm (take a break if you need to), then return your awareness to your horse.

○ **"STROKE" to begin and end a session**. Use very relaxed, softly molding hands. Glide over your horse's entire body with a light touch in a hand-over-hand motion. Stroke to wake up or sedate her energy, to give her a sense of wholeness, of where she begins and ends, and to gently introduce your touch.

○ **BEGIN TREATMENT in a comfortable zone**. Begin with gentle pressure where your horse welcomes it. Always work on the unimpaired side before proceeding to an area of pain.

○ **TOUCH PAIN with a warm palm and gentle patience**. Allow your horse time to gain confidence in your touch and movements, so that, when you reach a zone of discomfort, she may knowingly welcome you. Gradually work in this way toward a sensitive area, perhaps needing multiple sessions to desensitize it.

  You may aid an impaired area without touching it, by stimulating the movement of energy through the meridian running through it and its corresponding branch and specific area on the opposite side.

○ **APPLY PRESSURE gradually, HOLD 2–30 seconds, RELEASE SLOWLY**.

○ **PRESS from your center, in a natural, gentle, supportive manner**. The force for the pressure you apply, however gentle or firm, originates from your center. It travels to your upper back, on through the musculature of your shoulders and upper arms, and out through your fingertips or heel of palm. The force does not come from your fingers, hands or wrists; it passes through them.

○ **Press WITHOUT TENSION**. Your shoulders, arms, wrists, hands and fingers should be relaxed, flexible and sensitive. We often reflexively tense certain muscles in an effort to "do" something, rather than just allowing our knowing bodies to do it. We may also reflexively tense as our horses tense, especially when we are in physical contact with them. Tension inhibits our efforts, blocks the flow of energy that performs functions with ease. Bringing awareness to our own muscles in tension leads to their relaxation, and that of our horses. (Self-shiatsu techniques for relieving shoulder and hand tensions are given on pp. 26–29.)

○ **NEVER FORCE your horse's limbs**. Always "guide" them for manipulation, using a smooth, steady and rhythmic motion. Never force, never jerk, never rush. Don't work with a preconceived vision that you want to "push" toward. "Ask" for a stretch, a rotation, staying aware and sensitive to the range of motion. A **stretch** is done slowly and steadily and released slowly and steadily. The leg is fully, confidently **supported**, from the moment lifted until gently replaced on the ground.

○ **"JIGGLE" to relax and diagnose muscles and move energy**. Rock side to side or up and down, in a slow to medium pace, softly, gently, never with a rough feel or jerking motion.

○ **MAINTAIN PHYSICAL CONTACT** when you move from one side of your horse to the other.

○ **TAKE BREAKS** during treatment: to allow your horse time to move her own energy and make adjustments in response to what you have initiated, and to allow you to rest and recenter your energy. Stay with your horse during the break to keep a sense of continuity.

○ **INTERPRET RESISTANCE**. Too often a horse's apparent resistance is reinforced by the human response – the situation escalates, and understanding and healing are lost. We "dumb" humans, who don't speak horse and have lost the art of "listening", may not be seeing the pain or fear or instinct-based distraction at the root of the so-called "resistance". Your horse may move away from your helpful touch because: she's not in need; she's in pain – in that area or a proximal one; she remembers pain in that area; she's unhappy with your technique – perhaps you're too rough or abrupt or don't adequately support her limb; or she has other things/needs on her mind.

Respond with interest and patience. Observe. Don't give into frustration. To do otherwise would be counterproductive. The purpose of shiatsu is not to create more stress, but to relax and release the muscles so the energy will flow and rebalance. Observe your horse's "difficult" behavior as fascinating conversation, to be understood.

○ **BE PATIENT, EXPECT NOTHING**. Give yourself and your horse time to become comfortable and confident in these new ways of working together. Allow as much time as it takes. Hold no expectations. Make no judgements. If your horse doesn't want to give you a raised leg – don't insist, be content with whatever she will accept – pressure along the meridians, jiggling a stationary leg, percussion and moving muscle, rotating the opposite leg. The **intention of healing** allows it to happen.

○ **IMPROVISE: be creative!** The nature of energy is movement and change – don't get stuck in routines! Strive to be in the moment

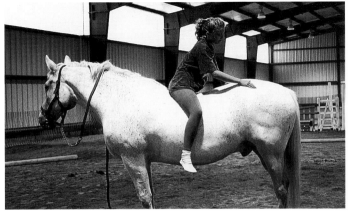

14.1 Improvise technique. *This isn't exactly what we'd suggest for the average rider, but the idea came naturally to these vaulters, worked great – allowing the leverage of dropped weight on hard worked muscles – and was welcomed by their deserving horses!*

each moment with your horse, in touch with her needs and your intuitive knowingness. Stay open to changing the sequence of techniques, adding some and eliminating others, and allowing your hands to improvise your own. (See Photo 14.1.)

Variables are multiple and common. Each horse is as individual in body sensitivity as in personality. Sensitivity alters with conditions and state of mind. There will be times when your horse may not want to give you her leg, or have her face touched, or her body touched — "Not now!" she says. Be flexible, and improvise your own variations of techniques that will work for you and your horse in the circumstances of the moment. (When Kate strained the hip-stifle musculature, I wanted to help the healing with leg rotations, but she would not let me — or our farrier — lift her leg for many months. We did a lot of improvising: we worked it resting on the ground and against my knee, learned to completely relax our arms to transfer relaxation and trust rather than confirm resistance, and she did her own leg rotations!)

○ **ENJOY YOURSELF**. Laughter, humor and playfulness defuse tensions, promote healing, and will take you far in a horse's esteem.

○ **THOUGHTS are energy** that direct us and create events. Be **without prejudgements**.

○ **SEE WHOLENESS**. See your horse as a bodymindspirit, a whole energetic system in want of balance, rather than as a collection of parts or a malfunctioning part.

○ **You are a CATALYST FOR HEALING**; the Ki energy within the patient heals.

15 *A Shiatsu Massage: Diagnosis and Treatment*

Stand or kneel near your horse in a receptive, not aggressive posture – a posture that says, "I'm here to listen and to gently help, if you need me". Let go of your tensions, let go of your "mind clutter", relax your shoulders, and breathe deeply and rhythmically from your center. Feel centered. Just "be".

Move your awareness to your horse. Notice if your mind or eyes linger on any particular area of her body: if they do, check this area during treatment for an imbalance in energy. Wait for a sign from your horse that you may begin – perhaps a nuzzle, a nudge, a deep sigh, a look or gesture (Photos 15.1a–c). When that sign comes (which should be within moments), quietly proceed.

Begin by stroking your horse over her entire body (see TECHNIQUES: Stroking, p. 78). Use the soft, light touch of your relaxed, moulding hands in a gliding, hand-over-hand motion. Work from the top of her neck toward her tail and down her legs, on one side, then the other. This introduction of your touch should give her a sense of wholeness, as you contact her energy.

Now proceed with pressure technique where your horse feels comfortable being touched. You could begin along the **Bladder Meridian**. Most horses should accept and enjoy being touched on this major pathway, except, of course, in areas of pain.

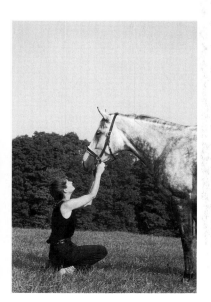

15.1a–c The sign to begin.

15.1a Pamela makes herself small and submissive to greet Katydid.

15.1b Katy greets Pamela.

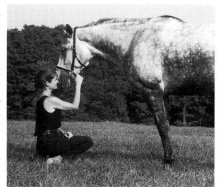

15.1c Katy yields to Pamela, as a sign that the session may begin.

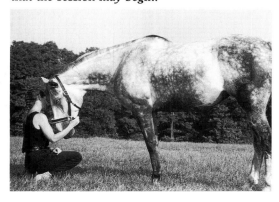

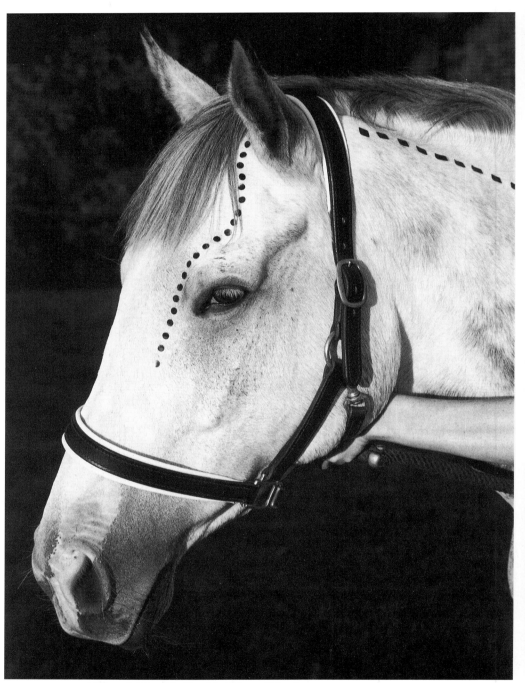

15.2a–d The Bladder Meridian of the horse.
15.2a

The Bladder Meridian (shown in Photos 15.2a–d) is the most important meridian for diagnosis and treatment. It is the largest meridian in
the body, covering the length of it, and is especially significant for the
back and spinal column. It connects directly with the other organ-

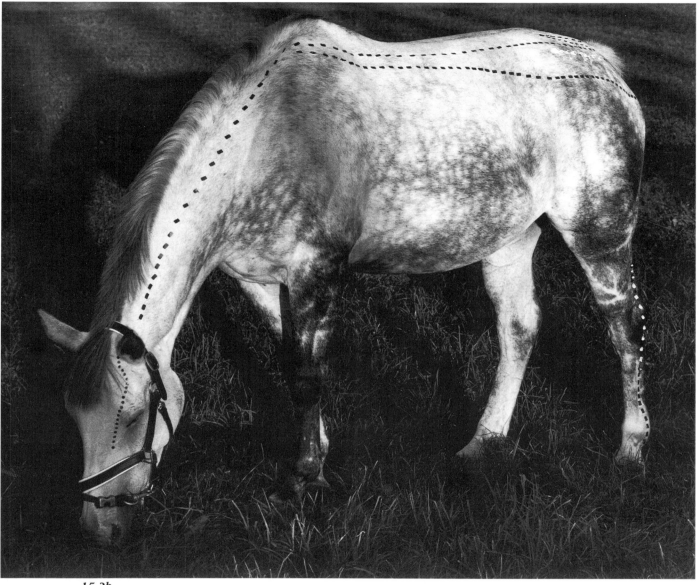

15.2b

function meridians, and has points used to diagnose and treat them as well. It is used for diagnosis/treatment when:

○ you want to assess the general health of your horse;
○ your goal is to generally rebalance your horse's energy for health maintenance/preventative reasons;
○ your horse appears to have a generalized malaise, but you are not aware of any specific problem;
○ you cannot identify the source of impairment;
○ you suspect a problem in the back and/or hindquarters.

92

TOUCHING
HORSES

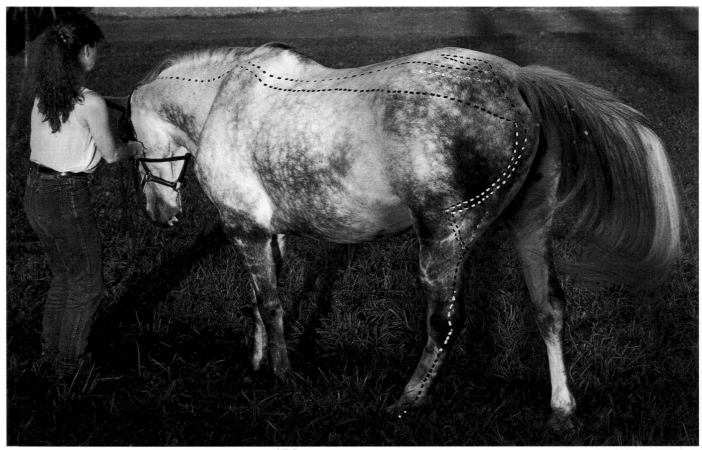

15.2c

When you diagnose through your touch, through the sensations received in your fingers and palms, diagnosis and treatment are one. As
your hands sense that an area is void of energy (kyo) or blocked with
too much (jitsu), they will simultaneously work to activate or sedate it.
Your hands will sense the general state of your horse's health as they
move and work along the Bladder Meridian to maintain or restore the
balance of energy. Shiatsu does not require a specific diagnosis.

The Bladder Meridian runs from the inside corner of the eye, over the
poll, along the neck — 2–4 inches below the mane root in the muscle
groove, over the withers on the dorsal edge of the scapula, along the
back — 2–4 inches below the protrusions of the spine in the muscle
groove — to near the end of the sacrum. It now zig-zags above back and
forth across the sacrum, then goes down the groove between the biceps
femoris and the semitendinosus muscles, passing close to the point of
buttock. It continues down this muscle groove, moving anterior toward
the lower end of the femur just above the stifle, then tracing the end
edge of the biceps femoris muscles to the end of the semitendinosus at
the posterior center of the leg. From here, it runs down the groove

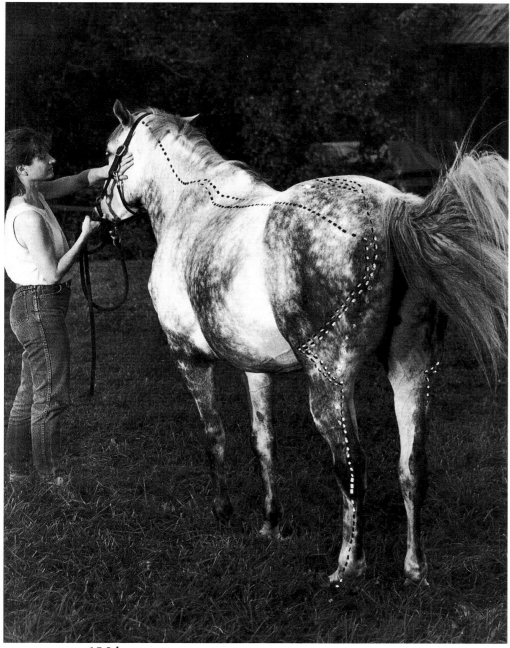

15.2d

edging the superficial flexor tendon, through the hock on the anterior edge of the tuber calcanei (point of hock), down the posterior edge of the large metatarsal (cannon) and pastern bones, to finally the outer bulb of heel of the foot. A second branch of the meridian begins at the center of the withers, just below the main branch. It goes to the posterior edge of the scapula, across the top of the ribs, just under the tuber coxae, across the pelvis to just before the main branch on its descent to the point of buttock. It now parallels the main branch just anterior to it, until they meet at the point at the terminus of the semitendinosus muscle at the posterior center of the leg.

The pathways of the major meridians tend to lie within muscle grooves, and many major tsubo points sit in anatomical indentations. Even the points of the foot are within subtle indentations. Knowing this makes the points and pathways easier to locate.

To find the Bladder Meridian, place your eight fingertips together on the edge of the neck crest or on the edge of the spine along the back; slide them downward, with light pressure, into the indentation of the muscle: this is where the main branch lies.

The proper position of your hands for palm pressure along this meridian is the natural position. If you lay a relaxed hand on the crest of your horse's neck, with your fingers draped over the other side, the heel of your palm will sit approximately over the line of the meridian, in the muscle indentation. The same position basically continues over the withers and along the back: your hands are relaxed over the spine, your fingers draped over the other side, the heels of your palms rest on the meridian.

We most often begin working the Bladder Meridian at the withers. This is because the association points to the other major meridians are located along it between the withers and the sacrum, and because maintenance of the back is so central to a horse's health. (Once you are able to readily sense energy imbalances, you will be able to very quickly assess your horse's general health by moving your palm over this stretch of the meridian — if you find heat and/or a void, you treat those points immediately, taking between thirty seconds and three-minutes to practice preventative care.) Position your hands side-by-side over the juncture of your horse's withers and back, with your heels of palms on the meridian. Let your hands mold to her body. Apply no pressure yet — just the weight of your relaxed hands. Check to feel that:
○ your tensions are released;
○ your shoulders are down;
○ your fingers and wrists are at ease;
○ you're standing balanced on the balls of your feet;
○ your breathing is slow, deep and rhythmic.
Gently lean weight (from your center) into the heels of your palms, applying a light to moderate degree of pressure: drop your weight vertically into the meridian through your moving hand (the one nearest your horse's hind end); apply gentle supportive pressure through your supporting hand. Hold for a few seconds, as you "listen" for "activity" under either or both hands. You may feel pulsations, faint or more obvious. If either palm feels the subtle sensation it's being pushed away, move on. Ideally your palms will feel pulled in, your pressure accepted, then a response under your moving hand — a gentle pulsing, the sense of energy flowing to and filling a silent space, or an agitated pulse slowing to a calm, even tempo. Slowly release.

The palm of your moving hand now slides about 2 inches rearward along the meridian. Both hands apply gradual pressure, hold, and release. The moving hand continues to move and work in this way through the sacrum (ignore the zig-zag over the sacrum). Your supporting hand will obviously have to move with you, before the reach of your arms becomes too distant and straining. Remember to keep your position comfortable, without tensions, while you're communicating through touch. Pressure will be light on your first "pass" along the back, as you warm the meridian and test for soreness and areas of kyo and jitsu. Over well-developed muscles, as through the hindquarters, slightly more pressure may be needed to contact the energy. From the sacrum, your moving hand works along the groove between the biceps femoris and semitendinosus muscles to beside the point of buttock, continues in the same indentation to just above the stifle, then follows the meridian as it angles to the back of the leg with the tendon, and slightly forward again down the groove of the superficial flexor tendon to the hock, approximately an inch anterior of the point of hock. You may stop here, at the hock, unless you feel that the lower leg needs attention, in which case you would continue to the last point on the foot. From the gaskin down, your supporting hand will work comfortably on the inside of the leg. You will also pause at closer intervals – about an inch apart – over this tendinous and bony area. (This whole sequence is depicted in Photos 15.3a–l.)

Unless you want to be very specific, such as for colic, do not try to find the exact location of tsubos (points) along the meridian: shiatsu's primary focus is on the flow of energy through the meridians, rather than on specific point therapy.

The length of time that you hold pressure will vary between two and thirty seconds. Your intuition and your feel of the energy will shape the rhythm of your work. In time, you'll gain confidence and adeptness in your ability. If you are unsure of what you are sensing, as all beginners are, hold for two to ten seconds, trust your intuition, and trust your intentions – you cannot harm your horse, and you are stimulating the healing process.

Remember to "listen", in both hands, to any sensation of energy, its quantity or lack of it. You may feel a "filling-up" of a "hollow" or still point – the energy moving to the kyo void: move on or, if you wish, continue to hold a moment longer and feel the movement of the energy. At times you'll feel energy pulsing under your supporting hand and no response under your moving hand's pressure: hold patiently for the energy to undam itself and reach the kyo point, or move on and recheck this area after you've done more work along the meridian. If your supporting hand senses being "pushed away", reposition it to where it feels "welcome" and comfortable for you both. Hold tight, "full", or over-energized jitsu areas until you feel them "relax", or your hand feels "pushed away". If your horse finds an area too sensitive for your touch, move on – when you return to the meridian with fingertip pressure, or return to the area later in the session, the blockage may have opened through your treatment elsewhere or a delayed response. You may

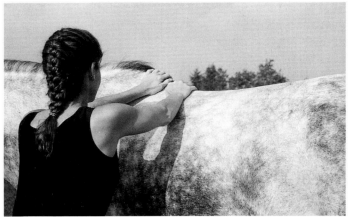

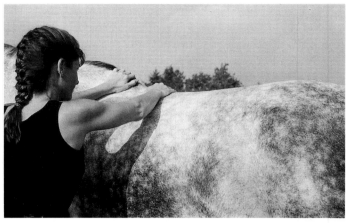

15.3a–1 Palm pressure along the Bladder Meridian.
15.3a A supporting hand and moving hand sit comfortably at the withers, with fingers draped over Kate's other side. Pamela gradually leans weight into the heels of her palms, holds for two to thirty seconds, and slowly releases.

15.3b The moving palm, in this sequence the right one, has moved approximately two inches along the meridian. Pressure is reapplied, held, and released. The palm then moves on. A rhythm establishes itself.

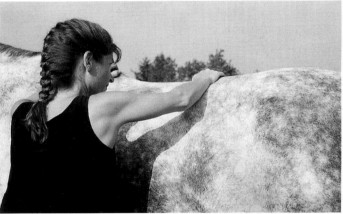

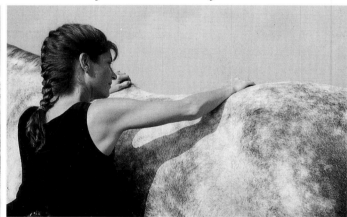

15.3e Her strength comes from her center, within her lower abdomen, travels through her upper back, shoulders and arms, and out through the heels of her palms.

15.3f There is no tension in her torso, shoulders, arms, wrists or hands.

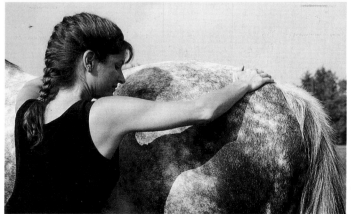

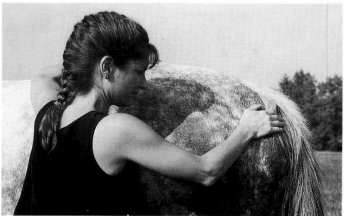

15.3i Her shoulders, arms, wrists, hands and fingers are relaxed, even though she exerts downward vertical pressure on the meridian where it is higher than her own shoulders. She is here on the muscle groove between the biceps femoris and the semitendinosus.

15.3j The meridian mainly follows the muscle indentations.

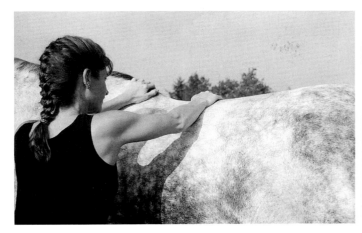

15.3c You can see from Pamela's arms, wrists and hands that a slight, but only slight, degree of pressure is used.

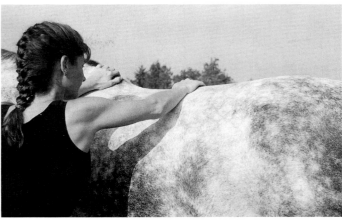

15.3d She gently leans and drops weight into her palms with her entire body, out of a balanced, stable base.

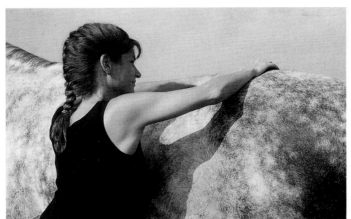

15.3g The supporting hand has moved over to maintain a comfortable, and supportive, position, not over stretched.

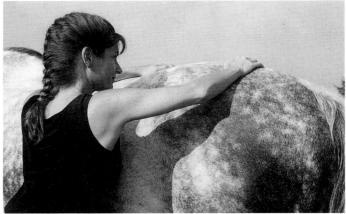

15.3h Through Katy's well muscled hindquarters, Pamela increases pressure slightly and holds for a few seconds longer at each pause.

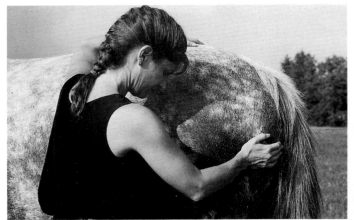

15.3k Pamela "listens" to the energy through her palm, sensing its flow or its lack and when to move on along the meridian.

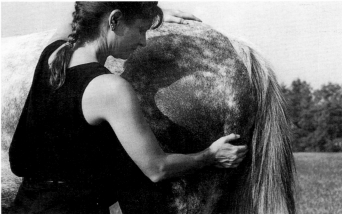

15.3l Pressure stimulates the movement of energy, activates or sedates it, summons it toward balance.

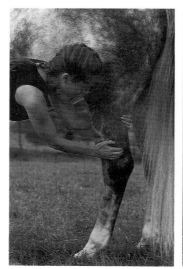
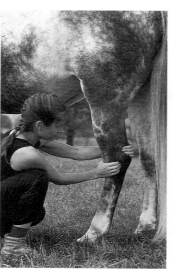
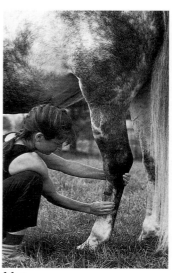
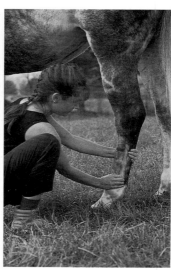

15.4a–f Fingertip pressure on the Bladder Meridian, lower hind leg.

15.4a With curled fingers, the four tips work as a unit to apply penetrating and sensitive pressure along the meridian.

15.4b Pamela's other hand supports from the inside of the leg, but note that the fingertips of that hand are still placed along the Bladder Meridian, listening to and affecting the movement of energy.

15.4c The meridian follows the lateral posterior line of the cannon and pastern bones to the outer bulb of heel of the foot.

15.4d On bony areas, as the hock and lower leg, use light, sensitive pressure, given mostly through the center fingers. We've omitted part of this sequence, but Pamela is pressing at approximately one inch intervals.

notice a communication between the energy under your moving hand and under your supporting hand, so that you, your two hands and arms and your horse form a circle of flow, a oneness. Eventually you will notice differing qualities in the energy and in its movement, you will sense a balanced flow from a "struggling" one and an over-energized one. This takes time and a trust in the process. It will come if you allow it to.

Palm pressure on one side of the horse is generally followed with fingertip pressure along the same meridian lines on the same side. Make a unit of the four fingers in your moving hand, curve them and drop weight in vertically to the meridian (the palm may lightly contact the horse's body); the palm of the supporting hand gently holds nearby. Along the back and croup, and over heavily muscled areas, use the muscles of your upper arm and back and the force from your center to apply pressure. Your wrist and hand are relaxed (not limp). Over heavily muscled areas such as the hindquarters, hold for a few seconds longer to sense energy and allow the penetrating benefit of your pressure. On the bony areas of the legs, press at closer intervals – every inch or so, with light, sensitized pressure. Pressure from the fingertips is more penetrating and active than that of the palm: it should be steady and firm, but comfortable (not too deep). Your fingertips, with their concentrated supply of nerves, are the most sensitive to detect energy, or its lack. (Photos 15.4a–f show fingertip pressure being applied on the Bladder Meridian of the hind leg.)

Once you have retraced the Bladder Meridian using fingertip pressure, move, while keeping contact with your horse's body, to her other side and repeat: first palm, then fingertip pressure, along the corresponding meridian lines.

You may now work with any known or suspect problem areas. Perhaps, before you began or during the session, your attention was drawn to a particular area. Or you found an overly sensitive point along the Bladder Meridian. Or your horse's movement has seemed slightly "off" in the hindquarters. How you now proceed will depend upon the existence and nature of any problem(s). You might work a few specific tsubos, or a muscle group, more meridian lines, or rotations and stretches of the hind limbs, for example.

If you have identified a specific problem, attend to it. Refer to the SHIATSU TREATMENT chapter for that body area, and to the "Index of Specific Problems". Work "around" overly sensitive or painful areas – refer to TECHNIQUES: Touching Pain, p. 73.

If your know or feel that an unidentified problem exists, work where your intuition or horse leads you. You will not hurt your horse by moving energy in an unneedy area, and you will stimulate her body's healing process. (**Note**: over-stretching or over-rotating stressed muscles, tendons or tissue can cause further damage, aggravate rather than help, so listen to your horse – if she resists, she may know something that you don't).

Horses often confirm the relief of pain or discomfort, that you have pressed in the right places, and that your healing touch is appreciated. Chewing, licking their gums, yawning, lowering the head and neck, and sighing, all signify relief and release of tension. Some horses hug, some kiss, and some say it all with large, grateful eyes. One stallion curls his neck to lower his muzzle into my hands for every sore point I release.

If your horse seems to have no problems and is still relaxed and attentive, you could work along the Bladder Meridian of the neck, if you have not already done so. You could add the other two lines of the neck, and the stretches. You could then, or instead, work the tail and stretch the entire spine. Stretching the spine is very beneficial to the horse, and is something they seem to appreciate. You may also work the shoulders and forelegs, and/or the hindquarters, doing a few techniques, only one, or an entire treatment. Be sure to take breaks if you and/or your horse need them, and stay alert to when you or your horse have "had enough" for the session. If you did not begin with the facial techniques, they make a nice ending, yet can be done at any time during the treatment.

As a last gesture, once again stroke your horse all over, to leave her with a sense of wholeness.

When your session is over, it is important to try to give your horse some time alone, so that she can focus, without distraction, on how her body now feels. Leave her in a roomy stall or, preferably, turned out alone. Try to give her at least ten minutes; thirty minutes or more is ideal. Observe her response, as she further readjusts herself, brilliantly expresses a renewed sense of well-being, or quietly absorbs the changes within.

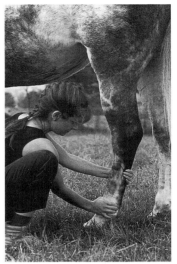

15.4e Pamela is squatting to the outside of Kate's leg, positioned to spring quickly off her toes. With an unknown horse or a known kicker, her position would be more precautionary.

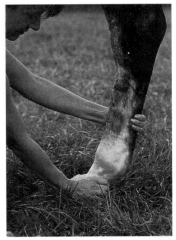

15.4f The fingertips press on the outer bulb of heel, the last point of the Bladder Meridian. With a few exceptions, shiatsu works meridians from head to rear, top towards toe, interior to extremities.

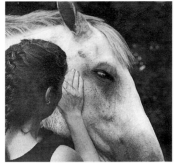

16.1a–b Moving muscle – the jaw.
16.1a Press, hold and release with your fingertips across the jaw muscle. Pamela here begins on the upper corner. Her palm rests comfortably on the large muscle as she works, adding warmth.

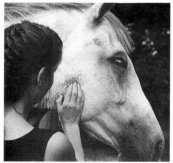

16.1b The hand keeps contact as you slide your fingertips over the skin from point to point at one inch intervals. The other hand gives supportive pressure on the opposite side of the head.

16   *The Head*

There's a good chance that your horse will learn to love these techniques, even pester you for them. My horses more often greet me with an ear or an eye for pressing than an exchange of warm breath – first things first, then kisses. Our pony, who came with our farm and a twenty-three-year-old habit of nipping and licking any and all human parts, now politely pushes his lip to my fingers to be rubbed and pressed. These techniques should keep your hands and your horse happily busy. They promote health, defuse old and unwanted habits such as mouthiness and ear or head shyness, yet take very little time. If your horse is head shy, proceed slowly, and also see "Releasing Tension at the Poll", p. 116.

The Jaw Muscle

Jaw tension is created by cribbing, tack or training problems, physical discomfort anywhere in the body, and emotional stress. These techniques, in conjunction with others, will help. It's best if your horse is not wearing a halter, which would conflict with your pressure and be in the way.

Moving muscle
(Photos 16.1a–b) Your supporting hand gently holds the other side of

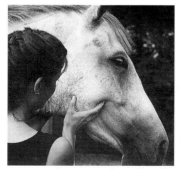

16.2a–b Front edge of jowl.
16.2a Mold your hand to the upper front edge of the jowl. Press your fingertips inward and up under the muscle. Hold for three to five seconds, release, slide downward an inch and repeat.

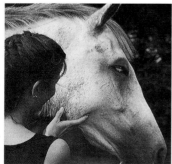

16.2b Continue down the full front edge of the jowl, without removing contact.

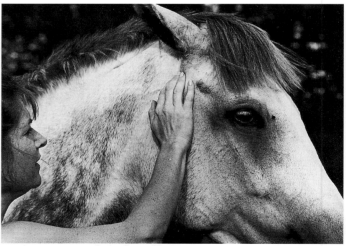

16.3a–c Posterior edge of jaw.
16.3a Begin at the top rear angle of the jaw bone, just below the ear. Pamela's three middle fingers press inward and slightly forward.

the face as you work. Place your fingertips on the upper corner of your horse's jaw, an inch or two beyond the outer corner of the eye. Press gently, hold for three to five seconds, release slowly. Slide your fingers downward, keeping contact, then press again, and so on. Continue across the whole cheek at 1-inch intervals, not removing contact.

Adding motion to your pressure will, in the case of the jaw muscle, be even more effective. As you press, push the skin upward, release, downward, release, sideways, release, to the other side, release, without removing contact. Each movement is about half an inch, and you must move the skin, not slide your fingertips over it. This is more specific and effective than a continuous circular motion.

Front edge of jowl
(Photos 16.2a–b) Mold your hand to the upper front edge of the jowl so that your fingertips press inward and up under the muscle. Pressure is applied gradually, held for three to five seconds, slowly released, slid down an inch or so, and repeated. This continues down the full front edge of the jowl.

Posterior edge of jaw
(Photos 16.3a–c) Fingertip pressure begins on the top of the rear angle of the jaw bone, just below the ear. Press inward, then slightly forward as though under the bone, hold, release and slide down about an inch to repeat. Follow the edge of the bone down as it borders the neck. Keep constant contact by sliding your moving hand over the skin between pressure points.

Once you've worked both sides of the jaw, mold your warm palms over them and quietly hold for a moment.

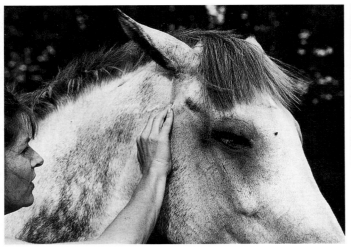

16.3b Her hand slides down without losing contact, presses in as though under the bone and holds for a few seconds.

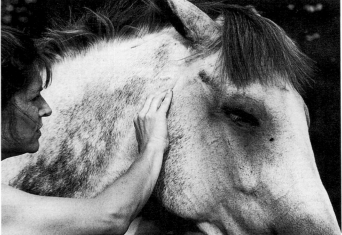

16.3c She continues at one inch intervals down the edge of the bone as it borders the neck.

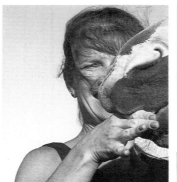

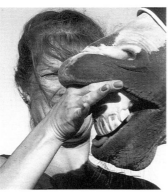

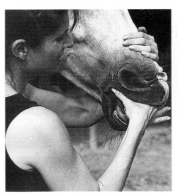

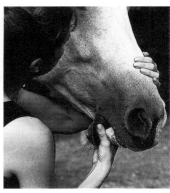

16.4a–d *The gums.*
16.4a *The web of your hand lifts your horse's upper lip.*

16.4b *It slides underneath the lip and onto the upper gum.*

16.4c *It then slides back and forth across the gum while pressing into it.*

16.4d *Repeat on the lower gum by pressing down and inward with the web of your hand.*

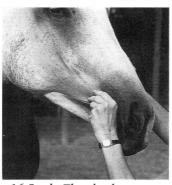

16.5a–b *The cheeks.*
16.5a *With the thumb against the inside of the cheek and the fingertips against the outside press towards each other and pull the cheek straight down towards the mouth …*

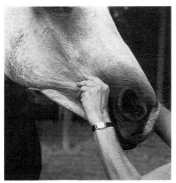

16.5b *… stretching the muscles. Pressure is firm, the hand is relaxed.*

Working the Mouth for the Gums and Cheeks

In many ways the horse's upper lip does double duty as a hand. It's a naturally active apparatus. And just as humans "speak" with their hands, so horses use this lip to "speak", sometimes of the stresses of domestic life. Points of the meridians are located on the upper and lower gums, and pressure there works to revive vitality and to defuse excessively mouthy habits. You should note that physical stress elsewhere in the body and/or emotional stress can be the base cause of unpleasant mouthiness – as long as the cause persists, it will seek an outlet somewhere. These techniques are beneficial for all horses, as a stimulant and release for the normally active mouth and the meridians running through it.

The gums

(Photos 16.4a–d) The web of your hand, between the thumb and index finger, lifts your horse's upper lip and slides underneath it onto the upper gum. It then slides back and forth across the gum while pressing into it. You can slide your hand five or six times if your horse is receptive. You may want to first wet your hand if your horse's gums feel dry. A supporting hand holds the head in a non-restrictive way. Repeat on the lower gum by pressing down and inward with your web of hand. You'll have to be more careful here to not jab the gums with the tips of your thumb and finger.

The cheeks

(Photos 16.5a–b) Insert your thumb into the corner of the mouth and slide it up so it's against the inside of the cheek – away from the teeth! – and your four fingers are flat against the outside of the cheek. Press your thumb and fingers toward each other as you pull the cheek straight down toward the mouth, stretching the muscles. Give firm pressure with a soft hand. Stroke two to four times before doing the other side. You can then repeat by alternating sides two or three times.

Yawns

(Photo 16.6) Stretching the cheeks usually stimulates a horse to chew, lick her gums and, often, yawn. This is a compliment to your technique, which you're also likely to get as a response to relieving pain, soreness and stiffness elsewhere in the body. Yawns are an especially wonderful response. A good yawn stretches and relaxes facial muscles as your hand can't do. The cheek-stretch actually taught my mare to self-stretch

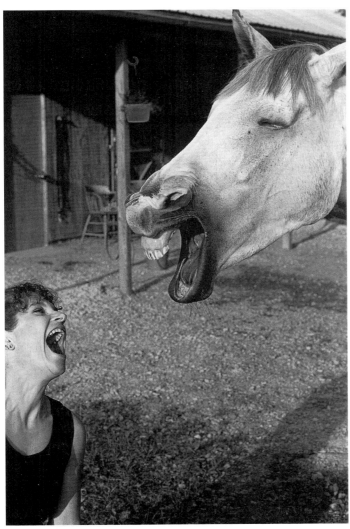

16.6 The yawn. The mouth techniques, particularly the stretching of the cheek muscles, always stimulate Kate to manipulate her facial muscles herself with huge, prolonged and twisting yawns that must feel great. Yawns seem to be contagious.

her facial muscles as she had not done before. Almost daily now she makes a series of huge, prolonged yawns that twist and exercise her face every which way. They obviously feel good to her. Some trainers are disturbed by a horse yawning when the bit is about to enter the mouth, but it pleases me as a sign of Kate's relaxation, acceptance and even pleased anticipation of our ride. The yawn is a preparatory stretch for work on the bit.

The Eyes

These techniques soothe and relax by using sensitive pressure on the bones circling the eye. They also stimulate the first points of four meridians (St, B, TH and GB). Begin at the outer corner of the eye, under the arched bone that extends back to the ear. Beginning on this bony protuberance eases the acceptance of touch to the sensitive eye (Photos 16.7a–b). Using your fingertips as a unit, or the edge of your thumb, gently press upward and directly into the edge of the bone. Hold for three to five seconds, slowly release, and slide your fingers half an inch along the bone to repeat. Follow the curve of the bone to the ear – under its final downswing is the joint of the jaw.

Move your fingertips to the lower inner corner of the eye. Press with sensitivity down on the edge of the bone of the eye socket (Photos 16.8a–c). Work this way along the lower edge to the outer corner, sliding your fingertips half a finger-width at a time.

The tip of the thumb is used to press into the upper edge of the eye socket. Beginning near the upper inner corner, place your thumb tip under the bone and your index fingertip on top of it. Press them very

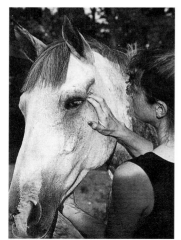

16.7a–b The temporal arch.
16.7a Using her fingertips as a unit, Pamela gently presses along the edge of this arched and curving bone. A supporting hand holds on the other side of the face.

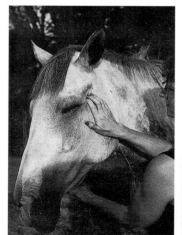

16.7b Pressure is directed up and in 90° to the bone edge. Just beyond her fingers is the joint of this bone with the jaw.

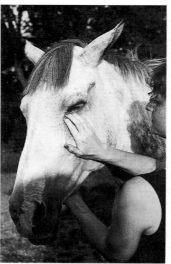 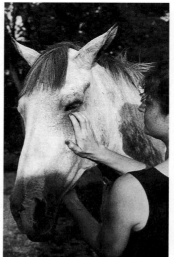 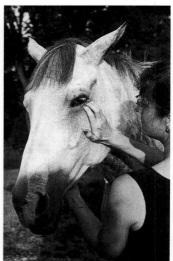

16.8a–c The lower edge of the eye socket.
16.8a Fingertips, working as a unit, begin at the lower inner corner.

16.8b Press with great sensitivity down and in onto the edge of the bone.

16.8c Press at one quarter inch intervals to the outer corner.

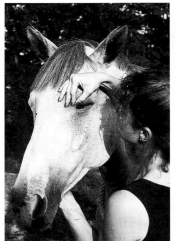 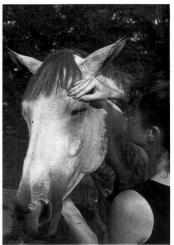 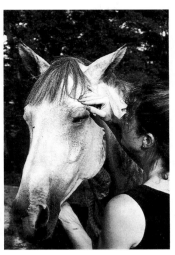 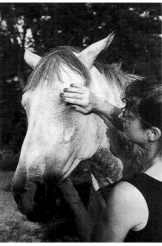

16.9a–c The upper edge of the eye socket.
16.9a Near the inner corner, press your thumb tip upward against the edge of the bone and your index fingertip softly down on it, as if lightly squeezing it.

16.9b The thumb gives most of the pressure, applied and held sensitively.

16.9c Slowly edge your way to the outer corner.

16.10 Finish the eye sequence by softly stroking your cupped hand two or three times over the eye. You may hold your hand there for a few moments to warm and soothe.

lightly towards each other, as if squeezing the bone. The thumb gives most of the pressure, firmly pressing upward, while the fingertip softly presses downward. Slowly edge your way to the outer corner – see Photos 16.9a–c.

Finish this sequence by softly stroking your cupped hand over the relaxed eye, from the inner to the outer corner (Photo 16.10). The fingertips move above the brow, the heel of palm under the eye: there is no pressure on the eye itself. Stroke gently two or three times. If your horse is very relaxed, hold a soft cupped hand over her eye without touching the lid. The warmth from your palm will soothe the resting eye.

These techniques work well on your own eyes, and are helpful for sinus and nose congestion. Doing them on yourself will give you a better feel for the manner and degree of pressure.

The Tearducts

The tearduct runs from the inner corner of the eye to the nostril, near its center, in an almost straight line. Clearing the duct of accumulated dirt and debris allows the tear fluid to drain properly through the nostril rather than pour excessively out of the eye. Try to locate the duct with your fingertips – you should be able to feel its subtle bulge under the skin.

Begin at the inner corner of the eye and work downward (see Photos 16.11a–b). Use a soft fingertip to lightly press and massage the duct by moving the skin over it in a chain of minute circles. Be sure to move the skin, not slide over it.

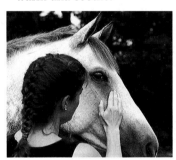

16.11a–b The tearducts.
16.11a Beginning at the inner corner of the eye, use a soft fingertip to press and lightly move the skin over the tearduct in minute circles.

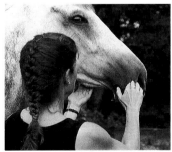

16.11b Pamela's pressure is so sensitively light that you can't tell she's working with her middle finger. Her pressure and circular movement are clearing the duct down its length to the nostril.

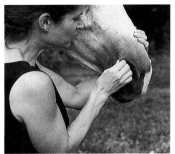

16.12a–b The nostrils.
16.12a The thumb and fingertips hold the outer flesh of the nostril, gently press towards each other, and lightly pull the flesh outward. Here the rim is gently pulled up and out.

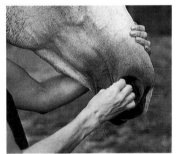

16.12b The nostril is now stretched outward as Pamela works her way around the fleshy rim.

The Nostrils

Gently hold the flesh of the nostril between your thumb and fingertips. Softly press as you also gently pull and stretch the flesh outward. Press and pull, hold for two seconds, softly release. Work your way around the fleshy rim, then do the other side (Photo 16.12a–b).

The Ears

Within each ear are tsubos that correspond to every part of the body, like a map. We use pressure over the entire ear rather than concern ourselves with the locations of these points. The tips of the ears are noteworthy for shock and colic. There are seventeen muscles that move each ear, and muscles of the neck attach near the base. Stretching these muscles and their attachments relieves tension associated with the head and neck, particularly the poll area, and helps to restore energy flow. If your horse is ear shy, you should also work the jaw and the techniques for relieving tension at the poll on p. 116.

Begin with rotations. Place your hand so the base of the ear is between your index and middle fingers (Photo 16.13a). Hold quietly for five to ten seconds to allow the warmth of your hand to soothe. Then press your hand downward as you move it in slow circles to rotate the ear. Circle in both directions about three times. This will help to relieve tension at the poll.

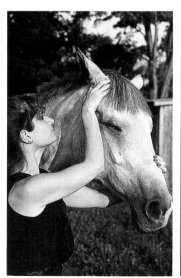 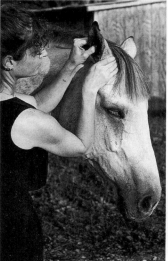 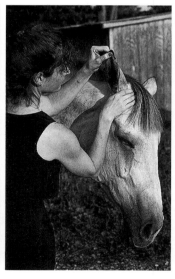

16.13a–f The ear.
16.13a With the base of the ear between the index and middle fingers, the hand presses downward and moves in slow circles, in both directions, to rotate the ear.

16.13b The thumb inside and the fingertips outside firmly press the ear between them. Begin at the base, but not too deeply in. The supporting hand holds at the base.

16.13c Work from the base up to the tip. Firmly hold the tip for five seconds or longer. You can continue to hold the tip as your other hand works up the other side of the ear.

Your supporting hand gently holds around the face. If your horse is relaxed and attentive, you can move this hand to hold one side of the ear base while working the other side. Both hands can then use alternating and simultaneous pressure on the same ear.

Use your thumb inside and your fingertips outside to gently but firmly press the ear between them. Begin at the base, but not too deeply into the ear (Photo 16.13b). Be very specific, with your pressure so that it's very clear what you are doing. Work your way up the side of the ear to the tip, pausing at half-inch intervals, holding for two to three seconds. Hold the tip a bit longer, with firm pressure (Photo 16.13c). Repeat two or three times, working near the edge and deeper in.

If both hands can work together, continue to hold the tip of the ear while your other hand presses up its other side.

Follow with alternate pressure from both hands (Photos 16.13d–e). Repeat as many times as you and your horse like. Keep working from the base to the tip on differing lines so that you cover most of the ear. You're pressing on the inside and outside of the ear at the same time, although you might switch emphasis. Kate usually lets me know which she needs by shifting her angle of presentation.

Use the thumbs and fingertips of both hands to firmly press and hold the tip of the ear (Photo 16.13f). Hold for five to ten seconds. As you hold the tip, gently lift the ear out from its base, stretching its muscles and those of the neck that attach by its base. This relieves tension in the area.

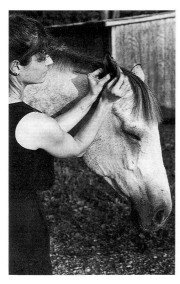

16.13d Both hands can then work together, alternating pressure up both sides of the ear. Repeat any number of times, working on differing lines to cover most of the ear.

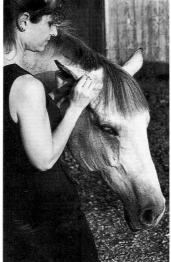

16.13e Press on the outside and inside of the ear at the same time, sometimes switching emphasis.

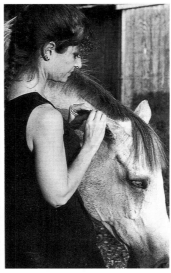

16.13f Press the tip firmly with the fingers of both hands. Hold for five to ten seconds. As you hold, gently pull the ear out from its base to stretch the muscles.

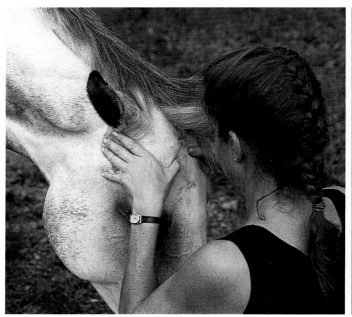

16.14 The forehead. Begin by pressing your thumbs side by side on the middle of the forehead. Alternately press, hold and release one thumb, slide the other thumb outward and repeat, and so on in a radiating pattern across the forehead. My hot blooded Kate is now so relaxed that she rests her nose bone and muzzle on Pamela.

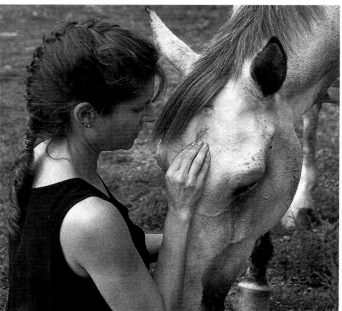

16.15 The "inner eye". The fingertips of her cupped hand softly rest on the centerline of Kate's forehead on the point called the "third eye" – the focal point of the "inner eye", the spirit. It's a quiet moment of being there for and with each other, a nice ending to the session.

Working the ears is relaxing and rejuvenating for the entire body. Work your own ears as well as your horse's, pressing all around the outside and the inner surface, pulling gently outward as you press. If you feel discomfort when you press on one part, continue to press firmly and the discomfort should go away. You'll soon know how good it feels. My horses think so.

The Forehead

Place your two thumbs side by side at the center of the forehead, allowing your hands to drape comfortably over the area above the eyes. Alternately press each thumb, holding for two to three seconds. Radiate your "walking", pressing thumbs outward from the forehead center. Move your thumbs sideways, upward and downward in a radiating pattern. Work with a gentle and slow press-and-release rhythm (Photo 16.14).

The point known as the "third eye" is located about one-third of the way up the center line of the forehead, just above the "brow". This is an important area. It is the focal point of the "inner eye", the spirit. It's said that this area can sense energy, and is the gate through which to calm the mind and reach intuitive knowledge. Soft fingertip pressure on your horse's "third eye" is a quiet moment between you, a moment of being there for and with each other (Photo 16.15).

17 *The Neck*

Sore, stiff and knotted neck muscles affect the way your horse moves. The muscles, ligaments and bones (the first seven vertebrae of the spinal column) connect to the head, the shoulder and the back (see Photos 17.1 and 17.2). Jaw tension, headaches, tight shoulders, sore and stiff backs and tail tension can derive from a troubled muscle or vertebral misalignment in the neck and from blocked meridian flow.

For general toning and specific treatment of the neck, we first use palm and fingertip pressure along three lines of meridians, to balance the energy, release the muscles and affect realignment of the cervical vertebrae. Pressure is also used specifically, such as to release the site of an injection or tension in the poll. We further relax the muscles and move energy with jiggling. The neck may then be stretched laterally, in both directions. If your horse is not tense in this area, nor through her head, you may use percussion, or you might jiggle the neck again. Remember that you can "reach" the neck by working the vertebrae and the Governing Vessel in the tail: if the neck is too tender or reactive to be touched, or extremely stiff, work with the tail before attempting to use pressure here. Rotating the fore and hind fetlock joints also releases excessive tightening within the neck by transmission through the meridians.

Pressure Along Meridians

There are six major meridians that flow through the neck, plus the Governing Vessel, which follows the dorsal median body line, and the

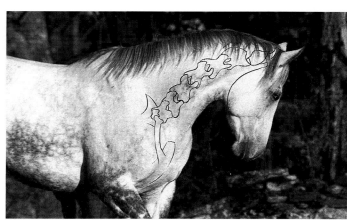

17.1 Cervical vertebrae.

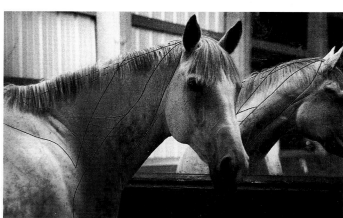

17.2 Major muscles of the neck.

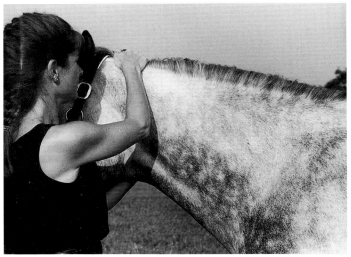

17.3a

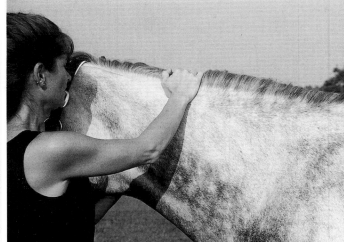

17.3b

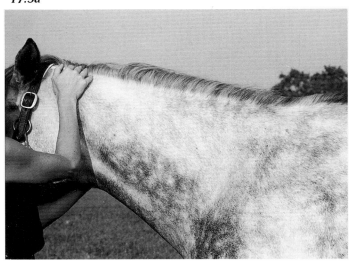

17.4a

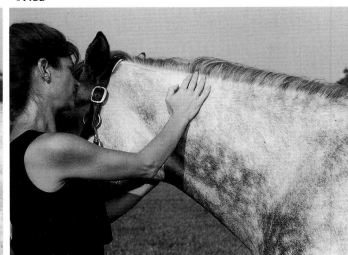

17.4b

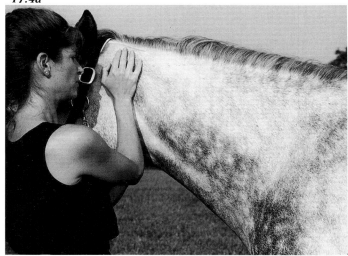

17.6a

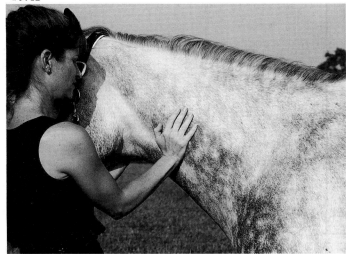

17.6b

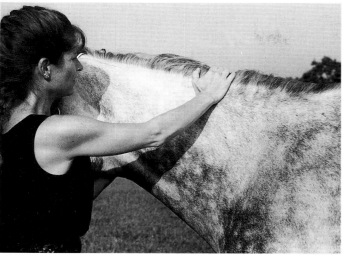

17.3c

17.3a–c The Bladder Meridian of the neck: palm pressure.
17.3a A supporting hand on the opposite side gives counter pressure.
17.3b The heel of the moving palm slowly presses in, holds and "listens", slowly releases, and slides an inch or two down the meridian (we've omitted parts of this sequence).
17.3c Both hands are positioned naturally and comfortably, molding to your horse's body.

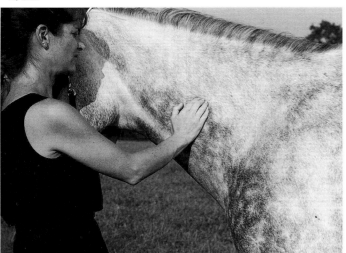

17.5

17.4a–b, 17.5 Center (spinal) line of neck: palm and fingertip pressure.
17.4a The moving palm begins centered over the first vertebra, with the little finger side of the heel pressing into the space between the joined bones.
17.4b Palm pressure follows the middle line of the vertebrae, directed into the space of each joint. You end the line at the joint of the last (7th) cervical vertebra and the first thoracic vertebra, with the edge of your heel of palm nestled comfortably against the shoulder blade.
17.5 Fingertip pressure on center line of neck. The four fingertips are used as a unit and sensitively mold to the contour of the bone.

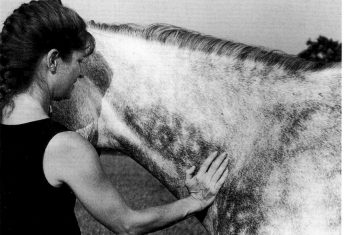

17.6c

17.6a–c Lower line of neck: palm pressure.
17.6a The heel of palm begins at the top of the jugular groove and presses upward and inward, with vertical pressure to the muscle. The supporting hand counters slightly higher, to oppose this pressure.

17.6b Pressure is on the muscle that follows the upper side of the groove, not on the vein in the groove. This line closely parallels the lower side edge of the vertebrae.
17.6c Follow this line to the shoulder blade.

Conception Vessel, tracing the ventral median line. The Bladder Meridian is the most useful for general diagnosis and treatment, and runs along the upper line of the neck, a varying few inches below the base of the mane. The Gall Bladder Meridian follows fairly closely below the course of the Bladder Meridian from the atlas (first cervical vertebra) to the top of the shoulder-blade. The Small Intestine and Triple Heater Meridians roughly follow the center line of the neck vertebrae. The Large Intestine and Stomach Meridians run closely, above and below the jugular groove.

Begin with pressure along the Bladder Meridian. Find it as you did along the back in the previous chapter, by placing your fingertips together at the base of the mane and sliding them downward into the indentation of the muscle. Your moving hand gives first palm and then fingertip pressure, beginning at the poll or as near to it as your horse will comfortably allow, and working to the withers. Look at the charts of this meridian (pp. 90−93) as it lies on Katydid, but remember that its location will vary somewhat as does each individual: Katy, for example, is fairly big-boned and broad; learn to feel for the meridian's location and trust your senses to find it. Lean your body's weight from your center into your horse along the meridian, first through the heel of your palm, then through your fingertips. Remember to give pressure at a ninety-degree angle to the body surface, and to "listen" for and respond to the energy. (See Photos 17.3a−c.)

Your other hand gives supporting counter-pressure on the opposite side of your horse's neck.

Work next down the center line of the cervical vertebrae. It's interesting how many people do not know where these vertebrae lie, but assume that they define the crest of the neck − which they don't! Begin again at the poll, working your palm down the center line of the bones (Photo 17.4a). Try to press the little-finger edge of your heel of palm into each joint between the vertebrae, and feel their lower and upper side edges with your thumb and middle fingers (Photo 17.4b). It's easier to feel their location when the muscles over them are relaxed. Jiggling may facilitate this. Fingertip pressure (Photo 17.5) should be made with the tips together as a unit, to avoid a poking sensation, and should also seek to press in the spaces between the bones. You are pressing to move energy, not necessarily to influence the position of the bones.

The lower line to work follows just above the jugular groove. Let the heel of your palm sit within the jugular groove and press it upward and inward at a ninety-degree angle to the muscle. Work this line from the jaw to the shoulder-blade. Your fingertips, like your heel of palm, should press on the muscle and not on the vein. As this may be a sensitive area, monitor your degree of pressure to your horse's response. (See Photos 17.6a−c.)

Jiggle the neck now, encouraging relaxation and movement, and noting the degree of movement. If your horse holds tension in her head, take care to use a fluid rather than a jarring motion.

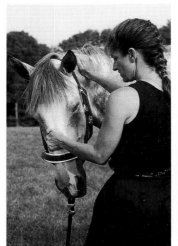
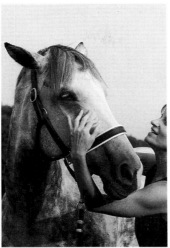
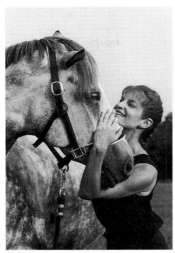

17.7a–c *Lateral stretch of the neck.*

17.7a *One hand begins to guide her head around into the bend as the other palm gently presses into the muscle at the top of the neck.*

17.7b *Once she begins to bend, Pamela readjusts the position of her arm and hand so she can comfortably continue to guide Kate's head around. She also moves her palm pressure a few inches down the neck.*

17.7c *She's using eye contact, as well as her voice, to coax Kate into a full and relaxed stretch. She stays close to the head, moving with it, guiding it while her palm pressure, moving progressively toward the shoulder, shapes the bend and exercises each cervical vertebral joint. Kate has stayed relaxed and attentive.*

Lateral Stretches and Flexion

To the degree possible, your horse's neck should be laterally stretched and flexed to both sides. Always work towards her easier side first. Work slowly and gently, never forcing or jarring, but encouraging her head to turn and her neck to bend to give the maximum stretch and flexion of the muscles and meridians.

Press one palm gently into the muscle at the top of the neck behind the head, on the side that will be flexed. Simultaneously move her head toward the same side with your other hand, with the flat of your hand on her face, **not** by pulling the halter (Photos 17.7a–c). Eye contact and a relaxed, encouraging voice may help.

Once she begins to bend, move the pressure from her upper neck a few inches toward her shoulder. Continue to coax her head around toward you as you apply pressure on the neck. Again, move your palm pressure 2–3 inches toward the shoulder, and bring her head around even more. Your progressive palm pressure works to exercise each vertebral joint as you "curl" her neck around (Photo 17.7c). If possible, continue until your palm pressure and her nose are near her shoulder-blade. You want her head and neck to remain low and relaxed throughout the exercise: if she tenses and raises her head, recenter and relax yourself and encourage her to relax before proceeding. Hold her maximum stretch for five to ten seconds. Bring her head back to an aligned position, supporting it throughout the movement, and repeat the flexion and stretch to the other side. Remember never to use jarring or thrusting motions.

If your horse doesn't want to have her head brought around into the stretch, there are two alternative methods.

Alternative technique 1: Flexing around you

Facing in the same direction as your horse, gently press the side of your head against her upper neck; place a moving hand on the opposite side of her face and a supporting one on the near side. Hold still, relaxed, for a moment. Now ask her to curl her head and neck around you, turning your own body to move with hers, and gently pressing your head and upper body against her neck. As she begins to come around, it may help your leverage to move your supporting hand to the withers. Continue to bring her head and neck around slowly until you've achieved the maximum stretch. Hold. Slowly release and bring her head and neck back to an aligned position. (See Photos 17.8a–c.)

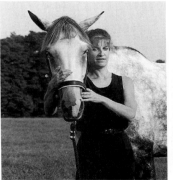 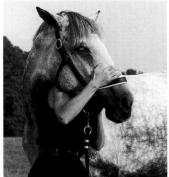 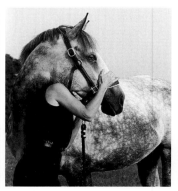

17.8a–c Alternative technique 1: flexing around you.
17.8a Gently press the side of your head against your horse's upper neck; a hand gently holds each side of her face. Hold still for a moment.

17.8b Ask her to curl her head and neck around you, turning your body to move with hers, always facing in the same direction as she is, and gently pressing your head and upper body against her neck.

17.8c Continue to slowly guide her head around until the maximum stretch of the neck is achieved. Hold this position for five to ten seconds. Release slowly.

Alternative technique 2: Stretching away from you

Face in the same direction as your horse, but on the opposite side to which she is going to flex. Place your moving palm on her near cheek and your supporting palm on the far side of her upper neck (Photo 17.9a). Slowly push her face away from you as you press her upper neck toward you. Try to keep her head and neck low. Avoid twisting her neck. Breathe deeply and exhale slowly as you lean your body towards her with your push, moving from your center. Slide your supporting hand down to mid-neck and push her face further away from you, into

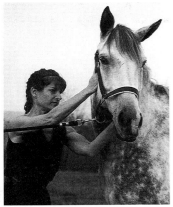
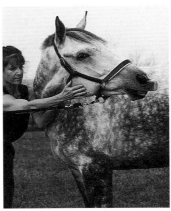
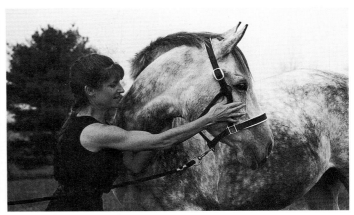

17.9a–c Alternative technique 2: stretching away from you.
17.9a With your palm on your horse's cheek, take a deep breath; exhale slowly as you lean your body toward her and slowly push her face away; at the same time, with your other palm on her far side, press her upper neck toward you. Try to keep her neck low.

17.9b Move your supporting hand farther down her neck as you continue to push her face away, creating as full a bend as possible with gently firm, not forceful, pressure. In this photo Pamela is not centered and has lost Kate's attention; Kate has responded with a mischievous expression of eye and lip and a tensing, resisting neck.

17.9c A moment later, Pamela recenters herself and Kate is again alert, relaxed and not at all resistant. Her middle neck is smoothly and fully stretched. Pamela will now release slowly.

the flexion (Photos 17.9b–c). Pressure is gently firm, never forceful. Stretch to the maximum, hold, and slowly release, bringing her head back into alignment.

You can now use percussion if you wish, and again jiggle.

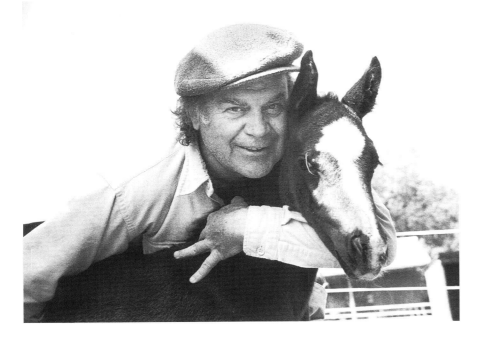

Young horses should only need loving hugs (Le Joyau d'Hiver at seven days).

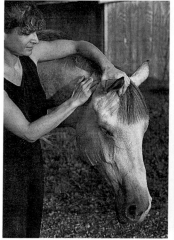 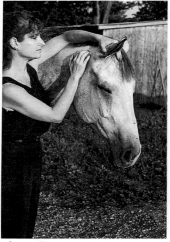 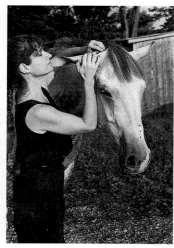

17.10a–f Releasing tension at the poll.

17.10a *Hold the ear forward, if your horse permits, with a gentle supporting hand. Begin with fingertip pressure directly behind the skull, between the first vertebra and the crest. Pressure is at first soft and increases gradually and steadily, inward, to the degree needed and tolerated. Hold for two to ten seconds. Kate is very sensitive in this area, but obviously welcomes the pressure and the relief.*

17.10b *Pressure is repeated on a slightly lower line, beginning near the upper caudal edge of the first vertebra. You can see in this photo the sensitive pressure given primarily with the two center fingertips.*

17.10c *Return to the base of the skull and gently press your fingertips into the space between it and the first vertebra. Holding the ear helps to open up the area.*

Releasing Tension at the Poll

The "poll" of the horse is the point where the back of the skull meets the first vertebra of the neck and spinal column, but the term is sometimes used to include the area above the first two vertebrae. The structure of these two bones allows for the independent up-and-down and side-to-side movement of the head. It is an area common to tension and sensitivity. The bad habits of a horse and/or rider, poor training techniques, and stress can add persistent aggravation. A horse who cribs, for example, will keep the muscles quite tight, possibly in spasm. The polls of head-shy and ear-shy horses are tense, a contributive if not original source of their shyness. Many horses will benefit from a regular release of the muscle tension and energy blockages that commonly build here.

If your horse is extremely sensitive and reluctant to be touched in this area, work the tail first, particularly the last vertebra of the tail, which relates directly to the first vertebra of the neck. Do the full spinal stretch (p. 148). Also work the jaw (p. 100) and the ears (p. 106). If your horse is still resistant, proceed as suggested in Chapter 12, "Touching Pain", beginning distally with tonification, slowly, patiently working toward the poll.

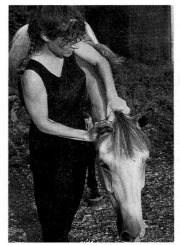

17.10d As Kate has relaxed
in response to the pressure,
Pamela uses her thumb to
press more deeply now.

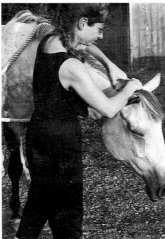

17.10e She walks her
thumbs down the length of
the muscle, as her fingertips
support on the other side of
the crest. If your horse
enjoys this, you can
continue to the shoulder.

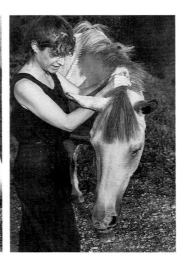

17.10f A soothing
completion: palms and
fingertips gently squeeze the
area behind the poll, hold,
and slowly release. The
palms send quiet warmth.

Begin on the less-sensitive side. Warm the poll area with your palm.
If it is very sensitive, barely touch the hair and hold for ten to thirty
seconds. Then proceed with specific pressure. If she'll allow you, hold
her ear forward with a gentle, supporting hand, to expose and open the
area. Place the fingertips of your moving hand behind the skull, between
the first vertebra and the crest (Photo 17.10a). Press gradually inward.
Hold for two to ten seconds. Slowly release the pressure. Press, hold
and release along this line below the crest at half- to one-inch intervals.
Repeat on a lower line, beginning near the upper caudal edge of the first
vertebra (Photo 17.10b). Return to the base of the skull and gently press
your fingertips into the space between it and the first vertebra (Photo
17.10c). Remember to be very gentle when you're pressing on bone.

If your horse is by now relaxed and enjoying the relief of your touch,
repeat down the length of the muscle with thumb pressure, beginning
close to the poll (Photo 17.10d). Thumb pressure is even more specific
and gives deeper release. Use the entire first joint of your thumb, rather
than the pointed tip. With both of your hands draped over the crest, you
might press simultaneously with both thumbs as your fingertips support
(Photo 17.10e). You might "walk" your thumbs along this line to the
shoulder, pressing into the muscle fibers.

A soothing completion to this treatment is to drape your hands side-
by-side over the crest behind the poll, with your heels of palms above
the vertebrae: squeeze the area gently, hold a few seconds, slowly
release (Photo 17.10f). Repeat the sequence on the other side.

18 *The Shoulders and Forelegs*

Shortened striding, a reluctant canter lead and being "off" are among the problems that can originate in the shoulder. Lower leg lameness is commonly caused by stress transmitted from a problem above. By the same rules, shoulder stiffness and pain can be a result, a symptom, of a problem elsewhere, such as in the neck, the back, the hindquarters, or a foot. If there is severe tightening, tenderness or pain within the shoulder, you should begin your treatment with the foreleg techniques, before using pressure directly on the shoulder. Working the forelegs activates energy throughout the shoulders, reaching the deeper muscles and releasing the muscles and joints.

Whether you are going to first work the forelegs or with pressure directly upon the shoulder, begin by using a standing-leg jiggle (p. 63), to give you a preliminary evaluation of the condition of the muscles and to initiate relaxation within them.

Six major meridians run to or from the front feet. The Large Intestine, Small Intestine and Triple Heater Meridians begin in the front feet and go up the outer (lateral) side of the legs to the head. The Lung, Heart and Heart Constrictor Meridians begin internally and go down the inner (medial) side of the legs to the front feet. There are two exceptions to this rule: the Large Intestine Meridian begins at the medial center of

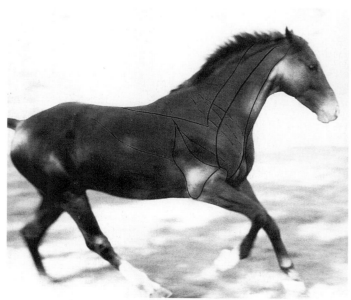

18.1 Muscles of the shoulder.

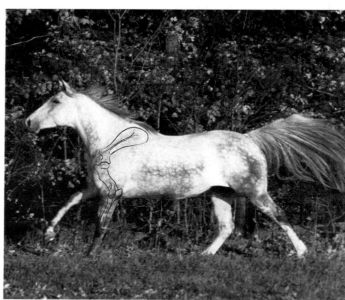

18.2 Skeletal structure of shoulder and foreleg.

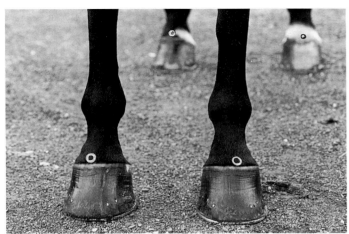

18.3a This tsubo point is about one quarter-inch lateral to the midpoint of the coronary band. The front pair are terminal points of the Triple Heater Meridian, the hind pair of the Stomach Meridian.

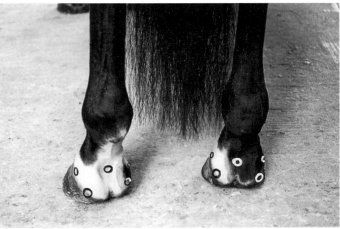

18.3b Meridian terminals of the foot. The locations are the same on the fore and hind feet.

the coronary band and goes up the medial side of the leg to the knee, crosses its front to the lateral side of the leg, then continues laterally; the Heart Meridian crosses behind the knee to run just lateral of the posterior center, and continues so through the pastern, then to the outer bulb of heel. Diagrams of the major meridians and descriptions of their superficial pathways can be found at the end of Appendix A. Photos 18.3a–b show the tsubo points of the foot, which are basically the same fore and hind.

Some key points of the forearm are shown for your general information in Photo 18.4. Photo 18.5 shows some key points of the shoulder.

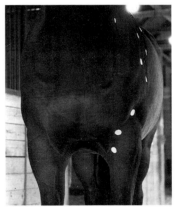

18.4 These three tsubo points are used to treat shoulder and elbow joint inflammation and myositis of the chest and upper arm muscles.

Pressure Along Meridians in the Foreleg

Palm and fingertip pressure is used along the meridians in the legs when the focus is on a medical rather than a muscular problem, but you may also begin here as a quiet way to move energy through the leg and shoulder. If there is too much pain in the shoulder for you to lift the leg, or too much pain in the other foot or leg to bear the forehand weight, work the meridians in the legs, then attempt rotations and stretches.

Within the form of shiatsu that Pamela practices, that developed by Master Shizuto Masunaga, the meridians are worked from the interior of the body outward to the extremities. So she generally works the meridians in the legs from above downward. (See Appendix A: Notes on the Twelve Major Meridians, YinYang Theory.) The palm warms the meridian to initiate healing, followed by fingertip or thumb pressure – they work sensitively with natural ease over the delicate structures of the legs. Remember to always use a supporting hand with your moving one. (See Photos 15.4a–f and 20.5a–d)

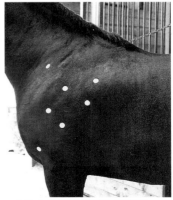

18.5 Some tsubo points relating to shoulder lameness and joint and muscle inflammation of the shoulder and elbow.

Rotations and Stretches of the Leg and Shoulder

Rotations and stretches of the leg primarily focus on muscular and joint problems, but also activate and move energy.

When you're working a raised leg, remember:

○ to gain your horse's confidence by your full and well-balanced support of her limb;

○ to keep the lower leg parallel to the ground;

○ to move your own body, your own energy, in order to move your horse's;

○ to replace her foot fully supported to the ground — never merely let go or drop it;

○ to switch sides often, so she doesn't begin to feel unbalanced.

Lifting and supporting the leg

Stand facing the front of your horse but to the outside of the leg that you're going to lift. Stand on the balls of your feet with a wide, secure base and bent, flexing knees. With one hand behind and above your horse's knee and the other hand over the lower cannon bone, lift her leg and raise it toward you (Photo 18.6a). With your upper hand supporting behind the knee, let your lower hand slide down to support the leg at the pastern. Slowly fold the lower leg upward until it is parallel to the ground (Photo 18.6b). In most of the stretching and rotation techniques, you want to work with the lower leg in this position, parallel to the ground. Now, keeping the lower leg in this position, gradually raise it

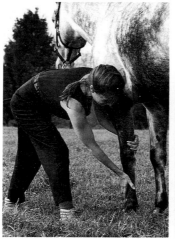 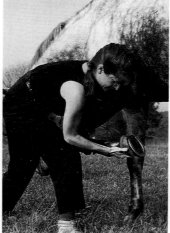 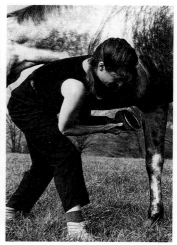

18.6a–c Lifting and supporting the foreleg.

18.6a Standing to the front and side, *lift* **the leg by placing one hand behind and above the knee, the other over the lower cannon bone, and raise the leg toward you.**

18.6b Fully support the leg by moving your hands to the knee and pastern, and raise the lower leg to a horizontal position.

18.6c Raise the horizontal lower leg gradually upward, so that you are closing the angles of the knee and the elbow, *stretching* **the muscles and joints through the shoulder, upper arm and leg.**

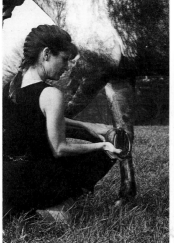 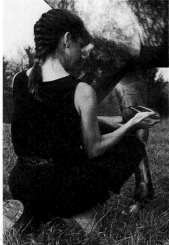 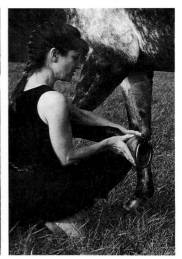

18.7a–c Hoof rotation and stretches.

18.7a Rotation. Kneeling with one knee on the ground, your other knee supports your horse's lower leg in a horizontal position. Your supporting hand holds the fetlock while your moving hand slowly rotates the hoof in either or both directions.

18.7b Stretch. Finish the rotations by stretching the hoof backward and forward. First fold the hoof up and in toward the fetlock, thereby stretching the muscles and tendons through the front of the leg.

18.7c Stretch. Now stretch the hoof forward and down by pressing your thumbs on the bulbs of the heel. Gradually increase pressure, like a crescendo, as you continue to support the lower leg in a horizontal position. Tsubo points are located on the bulbs of the heel where Pamela is pressing with her thumbs for the stretch.

toward the shoulder so that you are closing the angles of the knee and the elbow (Photo 18.6c). Do not force, and work slowly. If your horse is sore, aged or arthritic, you may want to raise and bend an inch or two, release a little, then raise a bit more, and so on, rather than using one fluid motion. Be sensitive to the point of slightest resistance, release a bit, and stretch again. Find your horse's limits, respect them, then gradually extend them.

Working the hoof and fetlock joint

Lower yourself to kneel with one knee on the ground and the other one raised. Support your horse's lower leg in the horizontal position on your raised knee. One hand supports at the fetlock while your moving hand, holding at the toe, slowly rotates the hoof two or three times in either or both directions (Photos 18.7a–c).

Complete the rotations with stretches: fold the hoof up and in toward the fetlock; now stretch the foot forward and down by pressing each of your thumbs on the bulbs of the heel, gradually increasing pressure while your arm and knee maintain the support and position of the leg. The points for treating tendon and joint inflammation are located on the bulbs of the heel.

From this kneeling position, jiggle the shoulder and leg.

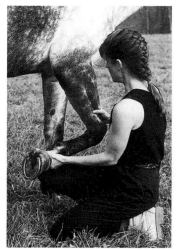

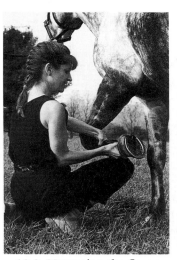

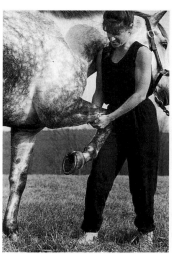

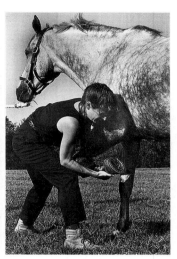

18.8 Massaging the forearm. Along the front of the forearm, beginning at the top and moving downward, gently squeeze your fingertips and palm towards each other to raise the muscle into your hand. Release, move down an inch or two and repeat.

18.9 Massaging the flexor tendons. Working from the knee toward the foot, gently press your thumb and fingertips toward each other, causing the tendons to rise into your warming palm.

18.10 Releasing the lower leg. While fully supporting just above the knee, gently tap the lower leg with your thigh, causing it to bounce softly. Tap about five times at one second intervals.

18.11 Rotation of the leg and shoulder. The lower leg should remain parallel to the ground throughout. Keep your body close to her shoulder to lend her a sense of support. Her leg should be relaxed and released to you. Rotate your entire body to rotate her leg. Begin with small circles, maybe six inches wide.

Massaging the forearm and flexor tendons

Again in the kneeling position, support your horse's leg horizontally to the ground with your knee and a hand holding firmly but gently at the foot. Your horse should feel that her leg is secure in its resting position. With the leg supported, the forearm muscles will be somewhat released and more receptive to therapeutic pressure. Along the front of the forearm, from the top down to the knee, use the pressure of your palm and fingertips, squeezing gently together to raise the muscle, release and move down an inch or two, squeeze again, and so forth (Photo 18.8).

Pressure upon the flexor tendons of the lower leg increases circulation and flexibility. Feel the tendons with the fingertips of your moving hand. Working from the knee toward the foot, press your thumb and fingertips toward each other. Be very gentle. Focus on warming the tendons with your palm as they rise into it from your pressure. Repeat on a line slightly farther forward on the lower leg, to press upon the ligament and muscle (Photo 18.9).

Releasing the lower leg

This technique releases and relaxes the muscles, joints and tendons of the lower leg. It is a good preparation for the rotations and stretches that follow. Raise and hold your horse's leg with both of your hands behind and just above her knee. Her lower leg will now "hang" loose. Place one of your legs out in front of the other and directly in front of your horse's "hanging" leg. Gently tap her lower leg with your thigh, causing it to softly bounce (Photo 18.10). Tap about five times at one-second intervals. Her foot and lower leg should swing freely in response to your movement. Such a response would indicate that your horse is relaxed, trusting and willing to continue. Support her foot to return it to the ground.

Rotations of the leg and shoulder

Raise your horse's leg. Support it with one hand behind and above the knee and the other beneath the pastern. Be sure to hold the lower leg parallel to the ground throughout the exercise. Begin, and end, with her hoof beneath her elbow, as in Photo 18.11. Your stance should be wide, your knees bent, your back straight, and your weight on the balls of your feet. Your outside elbow may be supported on your own upper leg. Keeping your body close to her shoulder will lend her a sense of support and encourage her to relax and release her leg to you.

Move your entire body to rotate her shoulder and foreleg. Move your body as a unit, shifting your weight from side to forward to side to back in a clockwise and/or counter-clockwise motion. Trace circles horizontal to the ground with your horse's entire leg. Do a few in each direction or in only one, if that feels right to you. Observe the amount of movement in the shoulder as you and her leg move.

The rotations are small to begin, perhaps 6 inches in diameter. They gradually expand in size, with the limit depending on your horse's degree of flexibility. You can include a few figure-eight patterns if it feels appropriate.

Replace your horse's foot on the ground, toe first, and move to her other leg – at this point, she may lift it and hand it to you. After working her second leg, do more rotations with both. You may find the joints and muscles more released on the second round.

Finish by jiggling each leg and note any increase of movement in the now released shoulder and elbow joints: they should feel and look freer, looser, relaxed, with perhaps a greater range of motion. The muscles should ripple as waves.

Inward and outward stretch of elbow

Support your horse's lower leg parallel to the ground, with one hand at her knee and the other at the pastern, as you kneel or squat beside the leg. Leaning your own lower arm or elbow on your thigh will give you further support. Use a soft, conforming hand but a firm arm movement to slowly push her knee inward, toward her other leg; you simultaneously draw her foot outward toward you; the elbow moves outward. Watch the degree of movement in the shoulder, upper arm and elbow. Stop when you feel resistance, and hold for a few seconds. (See Photo 18.12a.)

Now gently but firmly pull the knee back toward you and simultaneously push the foot, and elbow, inward, Watch the movement. Hold for a few seconds (Photo 18.12b). Repeat the sequence two or three times. Return the leg to its naturally aligned position, then to the ground.

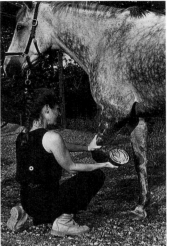

18.12a–b Inward and outward stretch of elbow. 18.12a Support the lower leg parallel to the ground and, perhaps, your own arm on your knee. With a soft but firm palm, slowly push her knee toward her other leg; you will simultaneously draw her foot outward **toward you, and, of course, the elbow. Push until you feel resistance, and watch the degree of movement in the shoulder. Hold for a few seconds before** ...

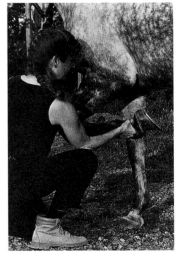

18.12b ... you pull the knee back toward you as you push the foot, and elbow, inward**. Again, hold a few seconds. Repeat the sequence two or three times.**

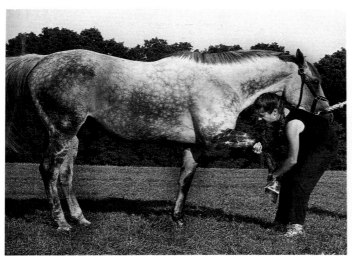

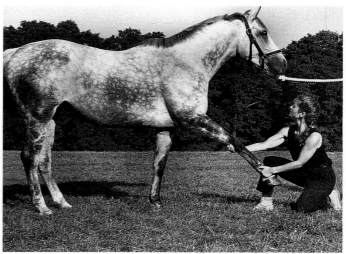

18.13a–c Forward stretch of foreleg and shoulder.
18.13a Hold the leg firmly and gently behind the knee and
pastern.

18.13b Stretch the leg long and low as you step and lean
weight backward. Use your relaxed bodyweight to make the
stretch, as you fully support the limb.

Full forward stretch of the leg and shoulder

Hold and support your horse's leg at her knee and fetlock (Photo 18.13a).
Step and lean your weight backward as you bring the leg with you,
stretching it out long and low (Photo 18.13b). Remember to move and
support from your center. Use your relaxed body weight and bend and
stretch your own legs and knees to stretch your horse's. Your horse's
response should be to relax and release her leg to you and to the stretch
– she can only do this if she feels fully confident in your support of her
leg and in your balanced movements. The leg is stretched forward and
downward. It should be stretched out through to the muscles of the
upper shoulder-blade, with the foot low to the ground (Photo 18.13c).
Stretch until you feel resistance. Release slightly, then stretch an inch or
two further if your horse permits. Hold for approximately five seconds,
or until she begins to "take back" her leg. Now fully release, slowly and
steadily, and replace her foot to the ground beneath her shoulder. After
stretching both legs forward, you want to flex and stretch the leg, elbow
and shoulder in the other direction.

Rearward stretch of the upper leg and shoulder

Still standing in front of your horse, facing her leg and chest, position
yourself to shift your weight forward, with one foot in front of the other.
Support your horse's lower leg horizontally to the ground. You may
position her knee on your thigh and your shoulder just to the inside of
her shoulder-blade. Slowly shift your weight forward, as if you were
lungeing, and use your weight, shoulder and thigh to stretch the joints
and muscles of her shoulder, upper arm and elbow rearward (Photos

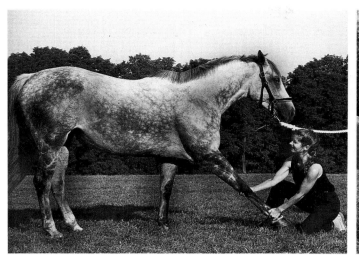

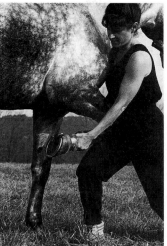

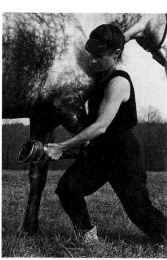

18.13c Stretch the leg toward the ground to its maximum limit, without forcing. Hold a few seconds. Release slowly as you return the leg to its standing position.

18.14a–b Stretching the shoulder and elbow rearward.
18.14a Position yourself to shift your weight forward, with one foot before the other. Position your horse's knee against your thigh, and support her lower leg horizontally to the ground. Now gradually push forward to stretch her shoulder and elbow joints and muscles toward her rear.

18.14b Move in a bit closer to increase the stretch. Stretch to the maximum limit. Never force. Release slowly.

18.14a–b). Move in a little closer to increase the stretch. Like a crescendo, stretch to your horse's maximum limit. Hold for a few seconds. Release slowly and steadily.

Pressure above and behind elbow

You're going to stretch the elbow joint forward to use fingertip pressure on the exposed and extended muscles above and behind it. Support your horse's leg between your thighs and with one hand behind her knee. Step backward with the leg to stretch the elbow forward. Use curved fingertips to press sensitively along the line of muscle rising from the elbow, beginning at the uppermost point (Photo 18.15a). Press, hold and release rhythmically, inching your line of pressure downward toward the elbow. As you press, simultaneously lean your body backward and gently pull her leg forward with your legs, your supporting hand, and your fingertip pressure – there will be a greater emphasis in the fingertip pressure. As you release the pressure, release the stretch somewhat by slightly leaning forward; slide your fingertips down an inch or two, repeat, and continue to the elbow (Photos 18.15b–c).

Pressure at inner elbow joint

With your horse's leg still supported between your own, press the web of your moving hand into the front of the elbow joint, in the crease

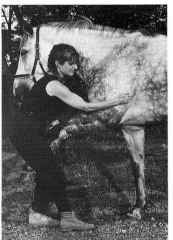 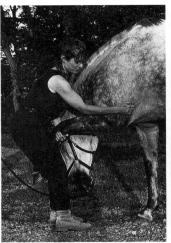 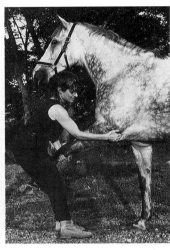

18.15a–c Pressure above and behind elbow.
18.15a Support your horse's leg between your own and with one hand behind her knee. Step backward to stretch her shoulder muscles and elbow joint forward. With curved fingertips, use sensitive pressure along the muscles above the elbow, starting at the top and working downward.

18.15b Press, hold and release rhythmically, inching your line of pressure toward the elbow.

18.15c As you press, lean your body backward and gently pull her leg forward. As you release fingertip pressure, release the stretch somewhat by slightly leaning forward.

between the upper arm and the forearm. With the web of your hand, your thumb and your index finger, apply inward pressure (Photos 18.16a).

Continue to apply pressure in this way down the muscle of the forearm. Press, hold, release, move on an inch or two and repeat (Photo 18.16b). The muscles should be pliable and more receptive with the leg in this position. Your horse should feel securely supported and relaxed.

Now jiggle the leg, to further release the muscles, joints and energy. To return her leg to the ground, support with both hands behind the knee, take a step towards her, release her leg from between yours, take a hold of her foot and place it, toe first, on the ground.

Downward stretch of shoulder and upper leg

Kneel with one knee on the ground and the other one raised to support your horse's lower leg parallel to the ground. One hand supports her pastern. Your moving hand, holding the front of her forearm above her knee, pulls her leg downward as you lean your raised, supporting knee towards her rear. Pull slowly to achieve a gradual stretch of the shoulder, elbow and forearm. Return your leg and hers to the beginning position and repeat the stretch, this time moving your leg and hers further rearward as you pull her forearm downward and back with your hand. (See Photo 18.17.)

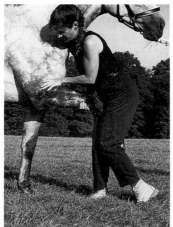 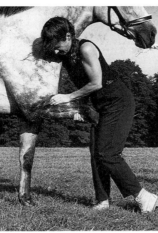 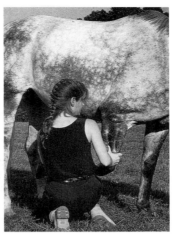

18.16a–b Pressure at inner elbow joint.
18.16a Supporting your horse's raised and relaxed leg between your own, press the web of your hand, your thumb and index finger into the crease between the upper and lower arm.

18.16b Continue the pressure at one or two inch intervals down the muscle of the forearm.

18.17 Downward stretch of shoulder and upper leg. A raised knee supports the horse's lower leg parallel to the ground. One hand supports at the pastern while the other, holding above the knee, pulls the leg downward. The raised, supporting knee tilts downward to assist in the stretch.

Jumper's stretch

Hold your horse's leg with both of your hands behind her knee. Slowly lift her knee straight up. At the first sign of resistance, lower the knee an inch or two, then continue to lift to the limb's limit (without force). Release slowly. (See Photo 18.18.)

Pressure on the Shoulder-blade and Muscles

Pressure along the front of the shoulder-blade

Routinely using deep pressure along this heavily muscled line releases tension where the muscles of the neck attach to the scapula. It is a common area of tightening, especially for jumpers (from the compressive impact of landing) and driving horses (from pulling).

To test this area for excessive tightness, first make sure that your horse's neck is relaxed, with the muscles coming into the shoulder released, not stretched or contracted. Then try to slide the little-finger blade edge of your hand under the shoulder-blade in two or three places. If your horse is uncomfortable and resistant, stretch and rotate the forelegs before proceeding here. On the other hand, if you are able to work the edge of your fingertips at least partially around the scapula, and your horse appears comfortable, then do proceed.

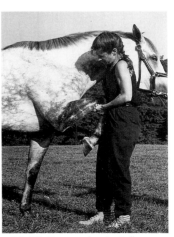

18.18 Jumper's stretch. Both hands support behind the knee and slowly lift straight up to point of resistance, release slightly, then lift to the limb's limit, without force.

Your supporting hand holds firmly at the withers. You lean your weight from your center toward the shoulder and into the fingertips of your moving hand. Your fingers are curved and pliant. They press into the muscle just in front of the scapula, beginning below the withers. The pressure is angled inward toward the shoulder (Photo 18.19a). As you

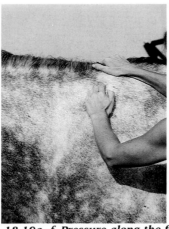
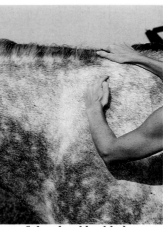
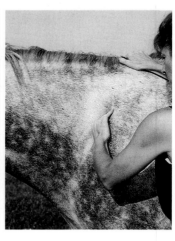

18.19a–f Pressure along the front of the shoulder blade.

18.19a Curved and pliant fingers press into the muscle along the forward edge of the scapula, beginning below the withers. Pressure is angled inward toward the bone.

18.19b As you press, slide your fingertips downward against the edge of the bone.

18.19c At this point your fingers should begin to work under the edge of the bone.

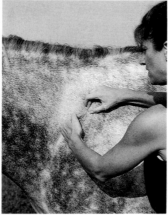
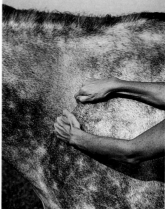
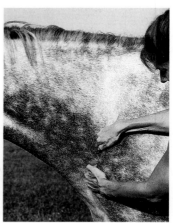

18.19d Move your supporting hand down to apply pressure alongside your moving hand.

18.19e Slide your lower hand down the scapula, press in, and hold. Now move your upper hand down to work alongside it. With both hands, press your fingertips in and under the edge of the bone, and hold with deep pressure to release the muscles. This point is a common area of tightening, especially for jumpers and driving horses.

18.19f Continue to press under the edge of the bone with the fingertips of both hands, inching one along, meeting it with the other, holding for two to five seconds, and so on down the full length of the shoulder.

press, very slowly slide your fingertips downward against the edge of the bone and use the blade edge, or side, of your little finger and fourth and third fingertips, pressing into the muscle toward under the bone. Hold for two to five seconds before sliding down an inch or two (Photo 18.19b).

At approximately one-third of your way down the front of the scapula your fingers should begin to work under the edge of the bone (Photo 18.19c). Once they do, move your supporting hand down to apply pressure along the side of your moving hand (Photo 18.19d). While your lower hand holds pressure, slide your upper hand down beside it to simultaneously hold pressure for a few seconds, then release your lower hand, slide it down a few inches, press inward, hold, release your upper hand and slide it down, and so on. Pressure is applied and released gradually. Avoid any poking movements, and be careful of your fingernails – avoid digging them in.

By midway along the front edge of the scapula of a healthy, relaxed shoulder, you should be able to press well under it, perhaps an inch or so (Photo 18.19e). Midway is also the point of the greatest tightening. Continue to press under the edge of the bone with the fingertips of both hands, inching one along at a time down its full length (Photo 18.19f).

A few leg rotations now will probably find a greater range of motion and flexibility in the joints. You can also repeat the use of pressure along the front of the shoulder-blade, if you feel it might help.

Resistance to deep pressure under the blade, persisting even after leg stretches and rotations, may be overcome by first using gentle pressure down its length, on both sides of the body. If your horse still resists, work on her neck, again if you're already done so, and include the lateral stretches; or work on her back and/or her hindquarters. Try once again to give deep pressure under the scapula, but *do not persist*. You may find that it has eased by tomorrow, or the next day.

Pressure along the rear of the shoulder

As your supporting hand holds at the withers, use the fingertips of your moving hand to locate the back edge of the scapula and the muscle indentation that drops vertically from it down to the elbow (Photo 18.20a). Use the blade edge of your fingertips to apply pressure down this line, pressing gradually into the muscle, holding, slowly releasing, sliding your hand down an inch or two and repeating (Photos 18.20b–c).

The pressure is given from your center, so there is no tension in your shoulder, elbow, wrist or hand. Pressure is inward and forward, as though you were trying to tuck your fingers under the muscle. As you move downward, you'll increasingly be able to do so.

When you can actually tuck the edge of your hand under the muscle, turn its blade edge so that you now press with the web edge, between your spread thumb and index finger. Use firm and deep pressure behind and under the muscle (Photos 18.20d–f). Slowly slide and work your hand downward to the elbow, increasing, holding and releasing the pressure every few inches.

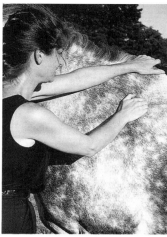 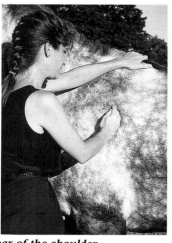 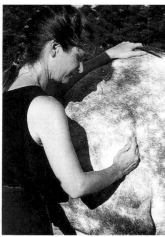

18.20a–f Pressure along the rear of the shoulder.

18.20a Locate the upper back edge of the scapula with your fingertips. The muscles form an indentation that drops vertically from this point to the elbow.

18.20b Use the blade edge of your fingertips to apply pressure down this line, gradually pressing into the muscle, holding a few seconds, slowly releasing, and sliding down an inch or so to repeat.

18.20c Pressure is angled inward and forward, as though to tuck your fingers under the muscle.

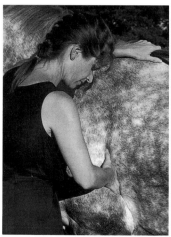 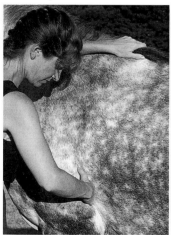 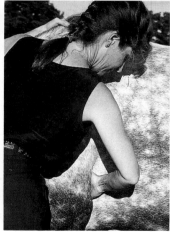

18.20d Turn the blade edge of your hand so that you are now pressing inward with the web edge. Press in and forward, now behind and under the muscle.

18.20e Press firmly and deeply as you slowly slide your hand downward toward the elbow, increasing pressure, holding for a few seconds, and slowly releasing.

18.20f Your horse may be sensitive near and underneath the elbow, and not allow this deep pressure at first. A few repeated treatments and the other shoulder/foreleg techiques should release and desensitize this common area of tightening.

19 *The Back*

The back is the unifying structure of the horse. It's defined by the spinal column. Contained within that is the central nervous system that controls most functions of the body. The longissimus dorsi muscles, the main muscles of the back, and the longest and largest of the horse, tie together the musculo-skeletal system: they attach to the last four cervical vertebrae, the shoulder-blade, the thoracic and lumbar vertebrae, the ribs, the sacrum, and the pelvis. The Bladder Meridian, the longest meridian of the body, traces the spinal column along the muscle groove of the longissimus dorsi, from the upper posterior edge of the shoulder-blade through the sacrum. This section of the meridian has association points with the other major meridians. A healthy back is clearly an important factor of a horse's overall health.

The design of the horse's back did not evolve to support a rider, nor to bascule over fences and invert on landing. It is a vital area very vulnerable to the stresses we put on it. An unbalanced or stiff rider, an incorrectly fitting saddle, an uncomfortable bit, improperly angled feet, an inverted neck carriage, uneven muscular or skeletal development, limb injuries, as well as over-stressed muscles, tendons, ligaments and joints, in the limbs or the back, will create back stiffness, discomfort and pain. A problem may be primary, say, back muscle soreness from over-exertion, or secondary, perhaps the compensatory result of an unevenly trimmed foot.

To fully treat a problem, you must eliminate its cause. It is important to evaluate the entire picture to determine the source of back stiffness and pain. This is not always so simple. The protective splinting that produces compensatory problems can leave a hidden trail. We examine the fit of the saddle, rider and training influences, possible emotional stress, trimming and shoeing of the feet, and any physical stress, including past injuries that perhaps haven't completely healed. We watch the horse move, allowing our eyes to be drawn to problem areas – the area that most strongly draws our focus is often the primary source of problems – the signs can be so subtle, and contrary to deductive reasoning, to be easily missed by those untrained in this way of working. Another technique we use is to move with the horse, imitating her movement as much as possible, feeling it from the inside out. (See TECHNIQUES: Evaluating Problems, p. 37.)

Whether a back problem is primary or secondary, it is often the first focus of treatment. We work through the Bladder Meridian, as described in Chapter 15, A Shiatsu Massage: Diagnosis and Treatment, from the withers through the sacrum. We would also work here to briefly evaluate and balance the energy in this critical area, for a general toning. We

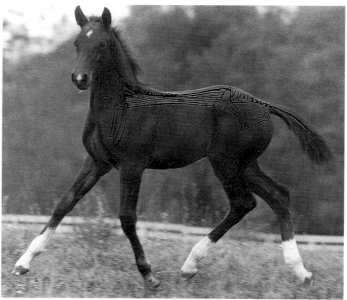

19.1 The longissimus dorsi muscles of the back and the spinal column.

feel along the meridian for heat and coldness, for dams of energy and empty silence, for jitsu and kyo, then seek to restore balance. We note any reactions to pressure: such areas may have heat, be jitsu, but could also be kyo, depleted, in need of energy. Palm and fingertip pressure are regularly used, but the thumb or elbow is sometimes wanted for increased specificity and intensity. The forearm gives a supportive and unspecific pressure to gently move energy in the meridian and muscles. (See TECHNIQUES: Moving Energy: Pressure, pp. 52–56.) A moving muscle technique and/or percussion may then be used along the meridian and the longissimus dorsi muscles, with small, close, quick and light movements.

Treating another area of the body may be what is required to relieve a back problem. Working the Bladder Meridian from the buttock to the hock is sometimes significant. Rotating the hind legs may release the back muscles, and the forward stretch of the hind legs may release the vertebral joints. Sideway stretches of the tail may help to increase lateral bend. All of the tail techniques promote suppleness through the body. The full spinal stretch through the tail is particularly good for the spine. Working the neck may prove to be the alleviating key. Pamela, in one case, was not seeing improvement of lumbar area pain, and was annoying the horse with her efforts, until she finally worked the neck – remember that the large muscle of the back connects to the last four cervical vertebrae. Remember that the back is the unifying structure of the whole, subject to the stresses of the near and distant parts.

Misaligned vertebrae are sometimes the source of back problems. They may be eased into alignment by working the Bladder Meridian and releasing the surrounding muscles. One or some of the additional techniques just mentioned might also be needed. A good roll by your horse might complete the adjustment. If you suspect a misalignment, and the problem remains after one shiatsu treatment (you should see improvement immediately, or at least within a few hours), consult a veterinary chiropractor.

If your horse suffers chronically from a back problem, possible sources of persistent stress should be explored with your veterinarian, farrier, and a competently observant ground-person.

20   *The Hindquarters*

The techniques that you choose to use on the hindquarters, as elsewhere, will depend on your horse and on the needs of the moment. It is generally a good idea to begin on the **Bladder Meridian**. You may next want to check the elasticity of the muscles by jiggling a relaxed leg or by softly percussing over the large muscle groups. If you suspect a problem within the pelvis/hip-stifle area, work the **Gall Bladder Meridian** that runs through it, and use pressure on the muscles and around the joints. You might then work one, two or three meridians in the legs. If your horse will safely allow you to lift and hold her hind leg, you might do rotations, then forward and/or rearward stretches, and/or rotations and stretches of the hooves. With the leg in a raised position, you could massage its released muscles and tendons. Percussing and jiggling would follow. Repeat techniques if your horse shows enjoyment and relief, and note the increased responsiveness of the muscles, joints and meridians.

If you know or suspect an area of sensitivity, remember to always work the opposite side of the horse first.

Pressure Along the Bladder Meridian

To treat the hindquarters, begin just above the tuber coxae, the bony protuberance that underlies the point of hip. Use palm and then fingertip pressure as described in SHIATSU TREATMENT: A Shiatsu Massage: Diagnosis and Treatment, p. 89. Work to the hock; you may want to do more

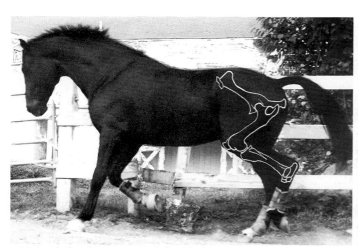

20.1 Skeletal structure of the hindquarters.

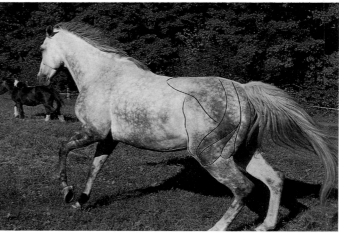

20.2 Muscles of the hindquarters.

meridian work on the lower legs later in the session.

A common point of soreness is the point of buttock (tuber ischii), in the indentation between the semimembranosus and the semitendinosus muscles, just posterior to a major corresponding point on the Bladder Meridian. When these muscles have been overworked, the point of buttock often wants deep pressure, such as from your thumb or your elbow. A horse will often even lean weight back into your pressure. Holding onto the tail *bone* with your supporting hand will give you more leverage to lean in your weight. (See Photo 9.2 on p. 55, the illustration of thumb pressure.)

Treatment of the Hip and Stifle

The Gall Bladder Meridian

This meridian is indicated for problems of the hip, stifle and hock, joints and tendons, and general muscle soreness. Its diagram is on p. 167. From the posterior edge of the last rib, it passes just below the tuber coxae, over the pelvis to the top of the hip joint, then to the great trochanter (prominence) of the femur. From there it follows close behind the posterior edge of the femur, passes through the stifle to an indentation centered under the head of the tibia bone (GB 34, a key point), then down the center of the tibia, down the center of the hock along the most prominent indentation, to the posterior edge of the metatarsal bones of the lower leg, more forward over the fetlock, down the lateral center of the pastern, to terminate at the lateral center of the coronary band. Work the meridian from the tuber coxae to the hock with palm, then fingertip pressure.

Some key tsubo points to use for sacral pain, and pain, inflammation and lameness in the hip joint and hindquarter muscles are shown in Photo 20.3.

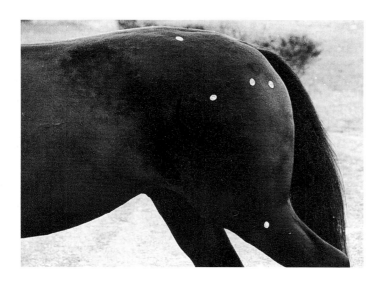

20.3 Some points used for pain, inflammation and/or lameness in the sacrum and hip joint and in the hindquarters in general.

Pressure Treatment of the Muscles

Begin with palm pressure just above the point of hip, on the gluteus maximus muscle, following the sequence shown in Photos 20.4a-l. Lean pressure into your heel of palm, hold a few seconds, slowly release, and slide your palm down an inch or two to repeat. Follow the muscle and pelvis down, from the top of the tuber coxae to the top of the hip joint. Now using the fingertips, repeat this line, pressing around the protruding tuber coxae bone, then down and in toward the pelvis and around the

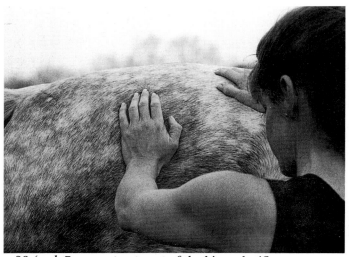

20.4a–l Pressure treatment of the hip and stifle.
20.4a Pamela begins with palm pressure just above the point of hip, on the gluteus maximus muscle, and follows the muscle to the hip joint.

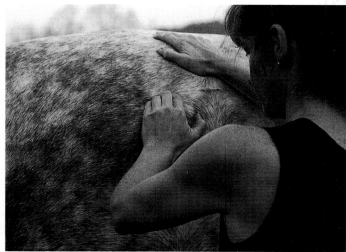

20.4b She next uses fingertip pressure around the protruding tuber coxae, pressing down and in at a 90° angle to the horse's body.

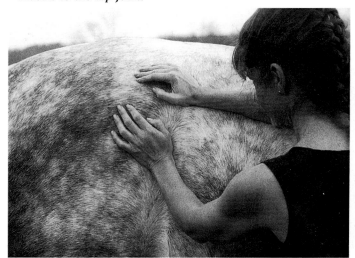

20.4e Both heels of palms press around the tuber coxae.

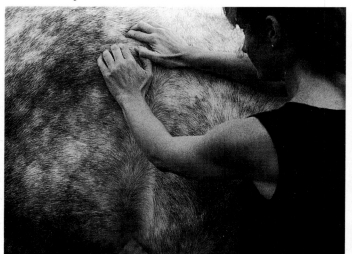

20.4f Then the fingertips of both hands press in around the bone.

top of the femur bone at the hip joint (which you may be able to feel under thick muscle). Next use palm pressure on a lower parallel line: press your heel of palm in around the sides and base of the tuber coxae, then follow the indentation between the gluteus and the tensor fasciae latae muscles to the base of the hip joint. Repeat with fingertips.

Now use increased pressure over the same area. Press with the heels of both palms around the tuber coxae, then with the fingertips of both hands. "Walk" your fingertip pressure over the gluteus muscle to the hip joint: your line of pressure follows the muscle fibers; your palms rest on

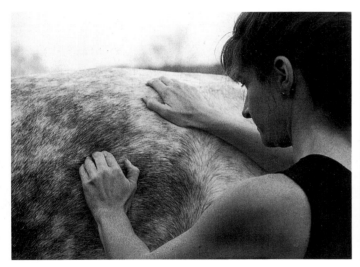

20.4c This continues along the muscle down the line of the pelvic bone to the hip joint.

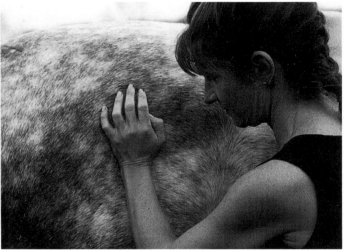

20.4d Now from under the tuber coxae she parallels her first line with palm pressure, following the interface of the gluteus maximus and the tensor fasciae latae muscles.

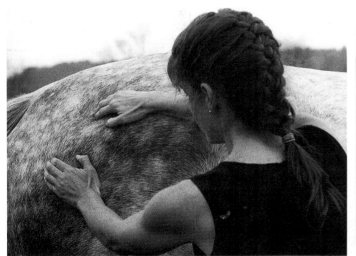

20.4g Fingertip pressure is "walked" down the muscle to the hip joint by advancing and pressing one hand at a time. The palms rest on the muscle comfortably.

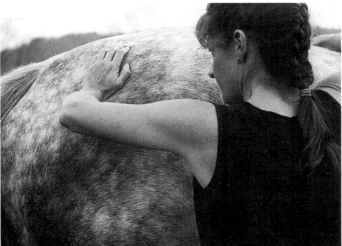

20.4h Deep palm pressure is now used on the muscles, following the direction of the fibers. Pressure is directed in towards the horse's center. Pamela keeps her own shoulders relaxed, widens the support of her other hand, and leans in from her center to gain leverage and strength.

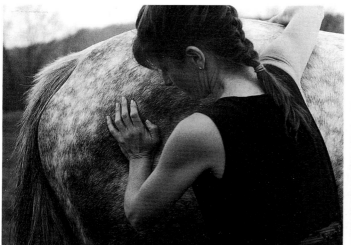

20.4i *The supporting arm applies opposing pressure, encouraging Katydid to not step away.*

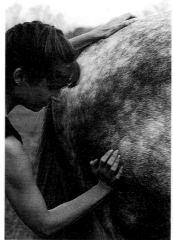

20.4j *Palm, then fingertip pressure are used following the indentations of the biceps femoris muscle from the hip joint to the stifle.*

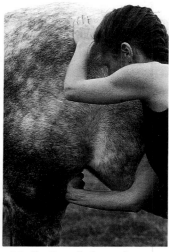

20.4k *Pamela leans in to apply palm and fingertip pressure together around the patella.*

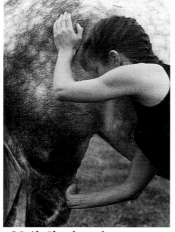

20.4l *She does the same above and below the stifle joint.*

the muscle to give simultaneous supporting pressure.

Work the gluteus maximus muscle above the pelvis with deeper palm pressure. Always follow the direction of the muscle fibers, from their attachment downward. When giving deep pressure, be sure to use opposing supporting pressure with your other palm and entire arm in this case, or the horse may step away. Support should always be "supportive", not forceful. Pressure is always applied gradually, held, and released gradually. A rhythm is established.

Do not use deep pressure, even over these large muscles, if your horse shows sensitivity. Instead, gently use the warmth of your palm, resting it over each sore area for as long as it feels right. You may also try the moving muscle technique. Rather than pressing directly inward at the usual 90° angle, you press obliquely across the muscle. Your line of pressure is across muscle fibers rather than aligned with them. You lean weight into your angled heel of palm so that the muscle bulges into your hand, then press in and down with your fingertips to pull the muscle slightly down. You repeat this two to four times across the muscle. (See p. 67, Photos 9.17a–b.) Your forearm and the back of your cupped hand give other gentle ways to "move muscle", as described in TECHNIQUES: Moving Muscle, p. 67.

From the hip joint to the stifle joint, you use palm, then fingertip pressure, following the upper and lower lines of the femur (the thigh bone). You work in the indentations of the biceps femoris muscle that covers this large bone. Use palm and fingertips around the patella and the lower end of the femur, then around the head of the tibia.

You could now use percussion over the hindquarter, and jiggle the leg to further release energy and check the state of the muscles. You might then proceed with meridian work on the legs. Or you might rotate and stretch the legs. After rotation and stretches, a repeat of pressure over the pelvis/hip-stifle area should find the muscles more yielding and the Bladder and Gall Bladder Meridians more "alive" with energy.

Meridians of the Hind Leg

There are six major meridians passing through the hindquarters to the hind feet. The Bladder, Gall Bladder and Stomach Meridians begin at the head, run the length of the body and along the outer (lateral) side of the legs. The Kidney, Liver and Spleen Meridians begin on the feet, run along the inner (medial) side of the legs, and terminate in the interior of the body. In general, the Bladder, Gall Bladder and Liver Meridians are concerned with mobility, the Stomach and Spleen Meridians with digestive disorders, and the Kidney, Liver and Spleen Meridians with problems of the blood, sex organs and circulation.

The locations of the Bladder and Gall Bladder Meridians have already been described. Descriptions for all of the major meridians and vessels are given with their diagrams at the end of Appendix A. The diagrams of the tsubo points of the foot (basically the same fore and hind) are on p. 119.

Three meridians are the most that you would normally work in one session, and one or two may suffice. The advanced practitioner, who locates the prime kyo problem, will focus on its governing meridian and

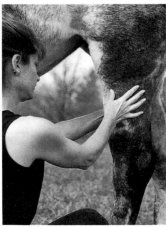 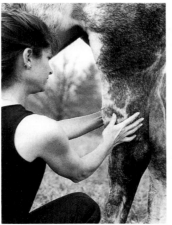 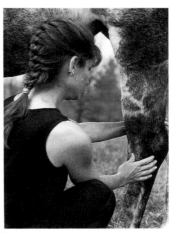 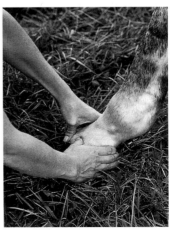

20.5a–d Stomach Meridian: stifle to hoof with thumb pressure.

20.5a This tsubo (St 36) on the Stomach Meridian is a general toning point, used to strengthen the immune system and build energy, and also used for stomach disorders, colic and lameness of the stifle. It's easily found – lying in the anterior depression below the stifle.

20.5b Pamela applies pressure by gently leaning her body weight into her thumb, not by "pressing". The thumb gives specific pressure with ease along this bony area. You could first warm a tsubo or a length of the meridian with light palm pressure – useful for a sensitive area.

20.5c The meridian from here goes to the anterior center of the leg, then straight down to the coronary band.

20.5d Pamela's left thumb presses on the last point of the Stomach Meridian: just lateral to the anterior center of the coronary band. It can be used for inflammation in the foot and constipation.

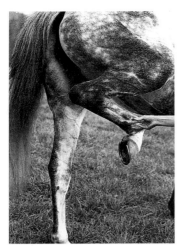

20.6 An unsafe leg to work with. Pamela has released and moved out of the way.

may also work its paired meridian and/or perhaps work a third corresponding one. The beginner may want to focus on one or two meridians at a time that seem to relate to the primary problem — e.g. the Bladder and Gall Bladder Meridians for hindquarter lameness, or the Stomach and Spleen Meridians for digestive disorders. (Photos 20.5a-d show thumb pressure being applied along the Stomach Meridian from stifle to hoof.)

Rotations and Stretches of the Hind Leg

Some horses will not relax and release their hind leg to you. With these horses, it's not safe to perform these particular techniques. If you have such a horse, work the meridians and the muscles with the techniques described above. Try to jiggle the hindquarters when she herself rests a leg in the tilted-toe position. If she won't allow this, try the standing-leg jiggle described for the shoulder. Try to desensitize the area as described in TECHNIQUES: Touching Pain, p. 73. If her resistance is not based in physical pain or its memory, energetic percussion over the large muscles might help — match your energy to hers (see TECHNIQUES: Quieting a Nervous horse, p. 71). Hopefully, as your horse learns to trust your shiatsu work and becomes familiar with the techniques, she'll entrust you with a safe hind leg. Remember that tension prevents healing — avoid pushing yourself and your horse into counter-productive, stressful and potentially dangerous confrontations. Don't feel frustrated. We weren't sure if my domineering Katydid would co-operate for the hind-leg photos without

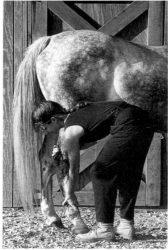 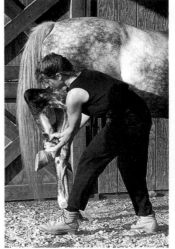 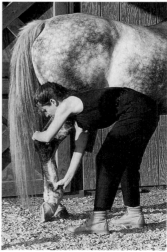

20.7a−c Lifting and releasing the leg.

20.7a Use both hands to ask for your horse's leg. Your knees should be flexed with weight on the balls of your feet. Lift with your lower body, from your center.

20.7b If she tenses, continue to gently hold (if you can safely do so) and allow her to release her leg into your relaxed, calmly confident, supportve hands.

20.7c Slowly lower the toe to the ground. Do not remove your hands or your support. In this position, the muscles of the limb are relaxed and ready for treatment.

dislocating Pamela's shoulder. (Notice that we move from the meadow to against the barn wall for the next sequence.) Kate actually does her own hind-leg rotations, but totally releasing the limb to my support and manipulation would be more beneficial. (See Photo 20.6.)

Lifting and releasing the leg

You must lift the leg with full support and control. Your horse must feel confident in your ability to support the weight and handle it comfortably, without you jerking, yanking, forcing or dropping it. Of course, make sure that she holds her weight on her other three legs – you are only to support one of them! Your relaxed hands, arms and body will send their message to your horse's limb.

With flexed knees and a wide stance, use both hands firmly but gently to ask for your horse's leg (Photo 20.7a). If she lifts it tensely, continue to gently hold and allow her to release it into your relaxed and sup-porting hands (Photo 20.7b). Slowly lower the toe to the ground without removing your hands or your support – you are responsible for that limb (Photo 20.7c). The muscles are now released into a relaxed state and ready to receive treatment. Jiggle, with one hand at the hock and the other softly holding the gaskin. Gently rock the leg back and forth as it pivots on the toe. Observe the movement of the muscles. You should be able to see them move around the hip socket. This technique will help to further release them, and should be repeated after the rotations and stretches.

It's very important to keep the horse's foot low to the ground for the raised-leg techniques. Raising a leg high compresses the muscles and vertebrae and can yank the hip joint, which explains why it even looks uncomfortable for a horse.

Rotations

Lift the leg and ask your horse to release it to your support. Support the pastern with one hand and the leg with the other and your arms and entire body. Keep your stance wide and your weight on the balls of your feet. Keep her toe near the ground (Photo 20.8). Move your entire body with her leg so that her toe traces small circles clockwise and counter-clockwise just off the ground. Move the leg rearward a few inches and repeat, still close to the ground. Bring the leg forward about 6 inches and repeat. Return the leg to its natural alignment and trace a larger circle. Repeat slightly rearward and slightly forward, still keeping the toe low. If you become tired, rest her toe on the ground for a moment without removing your gentle but firm hold. When you release, return the foot to the ground in its aligned position. The rotations begin small and increase to the size appropriate for your horse's size and degree of flexibility. As the size of circles increases, your speed slows. Do not force. Sometimes a small rotation or stretch is more beneficial than extending to the full range of motion, and sometimes one direction will help while working both directions may aggravate or be unnecessary – your horse will let you know.

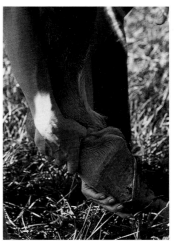

20.8 Leg rotations. Support the pastern with your hand and the leg with your arms and lower body strength. Keep the toe low to the ground. Trace small circles just above it by rotating your entire body with the leg as a unit. Move from your center.

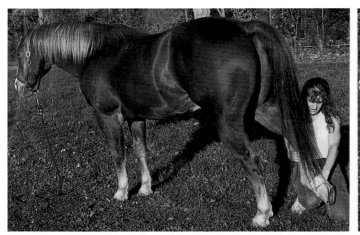

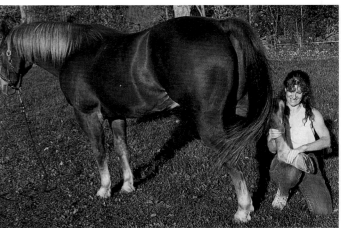

20.9a–c Leg rotation from kneeling position.
20.9a With the horse's flexed foot supported by your knee and hands, slowly raise and move your knee with your body in a smooth circular motion. Begin with your knee low to the ground.

20.9b Raise your knee and lean it rearward away from your horse.

An alternative rotation technique rests the horse's leg on your raised knee as you kneel. Lift the leg (from your standing position), have it released into your hands, kneel to the ground and rest the pastern across your thigh. Your two hands continue to support gently but firmly (Photos 20.9a-c). Slowly raise and lower your knee a number of times – this compression and release will relieve hip and lumbar tension. Now slowly raise and move your knee with your body in a circular motion, creating a smooth leg rotation. Begin with your knee low to the ground, raise it and lean it left or right, then up and around. Repeat in the opposite direction. Repeat in both directions a few times.

Rearward leg stretch

Take a wide stance with a straight back and flexed knees. Support the leg at the pastern and cannon, and remember to keep her foot low to the ground. Slowly shift and lean your weight into your front bending leg, lungeing forward (rearward to your horse). As you lean, bring your horse's leg with you, moving and stretching your body to move and stretch hers in a non-forceful way (Photo 20.10). Use your voice to encourage and praise her. You should both enjoy the stretch. Pause before resistance, release slightly, lunge and stretch again, leaning your entire body into it and stretching the leg to the limit of its range. Her foot is still low to the ground. Hold for a few seconds, so your horse can feel the stretch. Release before she pulls her leg away, so she stays relaxed and you keep control. Step backward with the leg and return the toe to the ground. Proceed to the forward stretch, or jiggle to observe improvement in the muscle tone and further release the entire hindquarter.

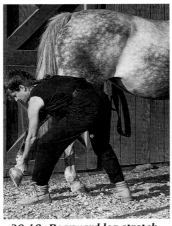

20.10 Rearward leg stretch.
Keep her toe low to the ground. *Supporting her leg at the pastern and cannon, lunge your weight forward bringing her leg with you. Move and stretch your body to stretch hers.*

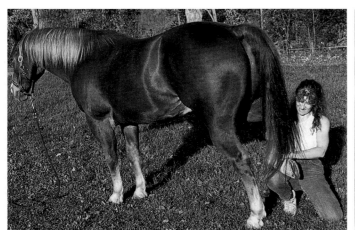

20.9c *Continue the circle by moving your knee up and around towards your horse, and then down. Repeat a few times, then in the opposite direction. Red, our aged Quarter Horse who's long backed and suffers navicular pain, is enjoying the increased attention to his hindquarters. This will in turn help to relieve his tendency towards forehand stiffness.*

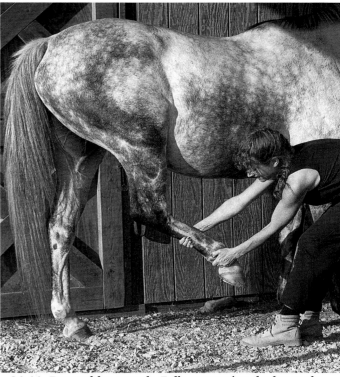

20.11 *Forward leg stretch. Fully supporting the leg at the pastern and cannon, and keeping her foot low to the ground, step and lean backwards. When you begin to feel a hint of resistance, stop and lean your weight back into your hips. Hold the stretch for a few seconds, then slowly release and either replace the toe to the ground or continue to the rearward stretch.*

Forward leg stretch

Still keeping your horse's foot low, support behind the pastern and cannon and step backward towards the shoulder. Keep your back straight and bend your knees. Lean back into your hips and let your weight help to stretch the length of your horse's leg forward (Photo 20.11). This also stretches out the Bladder Meridian. Pause before resistance, release slightly, then stretch to her maximum and hold. Release slowly and replace the toe under the hip. Jiggle, or repeat the rearward stretch.

It is generally best for the stretches to follow rotation. There are no rules about the order of these stretches, and they can be repeated twice. Complete them by jiggling.

Rotations and stretches of the hoof and fetlock

You can kneel and support your horse's lower leg on your knee, or stand if her attention span is short and she's likely to snatch her leg away. With one hand supporting the hoof and the other the fetlock, rotate the fetlock joint slowly in both directions three to five times. Feel the range of motion and increase it slightly with each rotation. Then

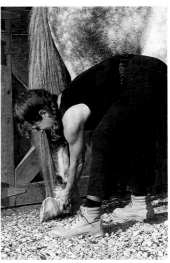

20.12 *Jumper's stretch. With her toe resting on the ground, press your thumbs downward on the back of the pastern. Press and release about five times with a slow and gentle bouncing effect.*

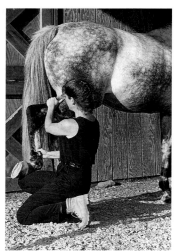

20.13 Massaging the tendons and muscles. Your knee and one hand support her leg as your other hand gently squeezes the relaxed tendons and muscles down the back of the leg, from the top of the gaskin to the hock. This encourages circulation and relieves stiffness.

slowly flex the joint by folding the foot towards the fetlock until you feel resistance. Hold for a few seconds. Release and slowly stretch the foot away. If you are supporting the foot on a knelt knee, press your thumbs on the bulbs of heel and gradually increase the stretch. You can repeat the stretches two or three times.

Jumper's stretch

Place the toe on the ground. Press your thumbs downward on the back of the pastern to flex the fetlock joint. Release. Do not force or use a jerking motion. Repeat five times, with a slow and gentle bouncing effect, slightly extending the limit with each press (Photo 20.12).

Massaging the Tendons and Muscles

Lift and support the lower leg, kneel, and place her flexed foot on your knee. Raising and lowering the supportive knee a few times, slowly, should reassure your horse that her leg is secure in this position. Continue to support with one hand at the fetlock. With your other hand, gently squeeze the now relaxed tendons and muscles down the back of the leg. Your draped hand presses its heel of palm and fingertips towards each other. Feel the tendons rise into your palm. Begin at the top of the gaskin and inch your way to the hock, holding for a few seconds at each pause. This warms the area and helps to relieve stiffness. Repeat two or three times. (See Photo 20.13.)

With the leg still in this relaxed, supported position, reach your moving hand up as high as you can toward the posterior of the buttocks. Bounce a relaxed fist off the hamstring muscles, inching your way down to the gaskin (Photo 20.14). Use the thumb side of your loose fist. Repeat two or three times. Fully support the leg as you return it to the ground.

These techniques can be done before rotation, if your horse is relaxed with the work. They can be preceded or followed by the hoof/fetlock movements. Jiggle if this completes your raised hind-leg work.

Finish your hindquarter work with percussion. If this completes your treatment session, use the stroking technique over the entire body to reunify the hind end and leave your horse with a sense of wholeness.

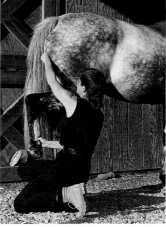

20.14 Percussion on the released hamstring muscles. While the leg is still supported and the muscles in a released position, bounce a relaxed fist down the back of the buttock to the gaskin. Repeat two or three times.

21   *The Tail and Spine*

Hidden within the magnificent fly swatter of the horse is the end of the spinal column, the last eighteen vertebrae. Along them are the beginning points of the **Governing Vessel**, which loops around the dorsal midline of the body, stores Ki energy and regulates its flow through the major Yang meridians and the central nervous system. Protected within the spinal column is the spinal cord, which connects to the brain to form the central nervous system. Pairs of nerves branch out of the spinal cord and exit between the individual vertebrae. Clearly, maintaining an aligned spinal column is important towards ensuring proper nerve transmission and a balanced flow of Ki.

The shiatsu techniques for the tail help to maintain spinal alignment. Exercising tail vertebrae sends a message up the spine of flexibility and flow. Developing suppleness in the tail works toward developing it through the body, including lateral flexibility. Through the Governing Vessel and the nervous system, problems are relieved along the spinal column, in the back and in the neck. The last vertebra of the tail relates to the first vertebra of the neck, and so on, and you can relieve soreness and stiffness in the neck by working with the tail. This is very helpful when the neck or the back is too sore to be touched.

Horses enjoy this work. They enjoy the stretches and the point pressure that moves energy along the spine. It's relaxing and imparts bodily awareness and a sense of wholeness. If your horse isn't comfortable being touched around the hind end or on her tail, and if there is a chance that she could kick out, work cautiously and introduce the techniques gradually. She should soon welcome them. A tight, tense tail should relax and develop good carriage. It may also make easy work of your veterinarian's next rectal palpation.

The techniques include arching stretches, sideway stretches, rotation of the individual vertebrae, point pressure, and a full spinal stretch.

Tail Stretches

Arching stretches

Take your horse's tail from underneath with both hands close together, your upper hand a few inches below the dock. The palm of the upper hand gently, firmly and slowly pushes the tail upward to form a wide arch. The lower supporting hand gently holds (Photo 21.1a). Do not arch the tail so much that wrinkles form at the dock, compressing the vertebrae adjacent to the ones you're releasing. Hold for three to five

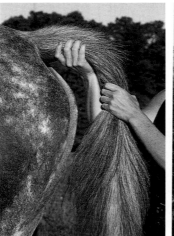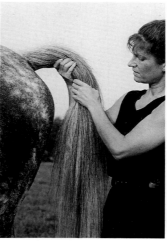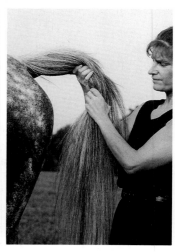

*21.1a–c Arching stretches.
21.1a With both hands
close together, the palm of
your upper hand presses the
tail upward to form a gentle
arch. An extreme arch
would cause unwanted
compression at the root and
the adjacent vertebrae.*

*21.1b Repeat every few
inches, holding for three to
five seconds.*

*21.1c Work to midway
down the tail.*

seconds. Relax the tail downward, slide your hands down a few inches, and repeat (Photos 21.1b-c). Continue to about midway down the tail bones.

Sideway stretches

One hand holds below the dock, the other over the last vertebrae. Raise the tail with both hands, but do not raise it above its natural alignment with the body – Photo 21.2 shows the wrong way. Slowly walk it to one side until you reach the buttock (Photo 21.3), hold a moment as you slightly pull sideways, walk it back and to the other side, hold and lightly pull, walk it back and return it to its natural lowered and centered position – don't just drop it. It is very important that you move the tail with both hands holding the vertebrae and by walking with it, not by just moving your arms. You need to move your energy in order to move your horse's, and it is much more supportive if your energy moves in concert with hers.

Pamela has found the sideway stretches particularly helpful in increasing a horse's lateral bend.

Rotation of Individual Vertebrae

Isolate each vertebra by first finding its upper joint. Using your thumbs and fingertips, hold the upper bone with one hand while the lower thumb presses into the joint for a few seconds. Then slowly and carefully rotate the lower section, gently flexing it in each direction to draw a small circle. This should relieve tension and alleviate kinks. Begin at the top of the tail and work your way downward, working each vertebra and joint in turn (Photo 21.4).

Point Pressure

Working the Governing Vessel is optional. There are times when it may be the only technique you use. You may intuitively work there in a moment of need, as a way to reach untouchable pain or an otherwise unresponsive problem, as a continuation of work along the spine through the Bladder Meridian, or while working with the tail.

The first point of this pathway lies in the hollow of the underside of the tail at its root. There is another point at the tip of the tail, on the last vertebra, which you might use to rebalance energy through the spine.

You can move energy down the tail by beginning fingertip pressure on the underside of the root, in the hollow, and continuing down to the tip. A supporting hand holds along the vertebrae, raising the tail enough to allow you to work underneath. The fingertips of the supporting hand feel the response of the energy along the pathway.

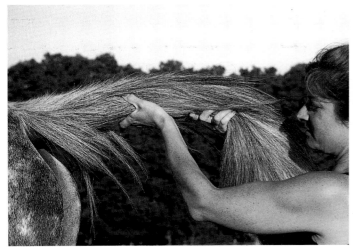

21.2 The wrong way to lift the tail. This way compresses the vertebrae at the dock and interrupts the flow of energy and nerve transmissions. Instead, hold the tail at a low angle that creates a natural and relaxed continuation of the spine, so your horse will get the full benefit of the stretches and avoid tension.

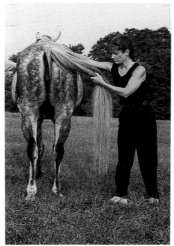

21.3 Sideway stretches. From this view you can see a good angle for the tail. With both hands lifting and holding the tail bone, slowly walk it to one side until you reach the buttock, then walk it to the other side, then return it to its natural, lowered place.

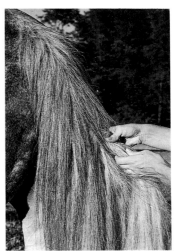

21.4 Rotation of individual vertebrae. Using thumbs and fingertips, hold adjacent bones, gently but firmly press your thumb into the joint, then very slowly rotate the lower section. Work down the tail.

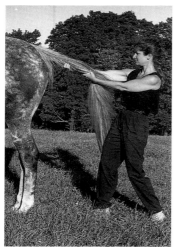

21.5 Full spinal stretch. Both hands hold the tail bone smoothly aligned and straight to the rest of the spine. With your arms and back straight, lean all of your weight backward into a bending leg. Your horse should respond by pulling straight away from you to create a full spinal stretch. Hold five to ten seconds before slowly releasing.

Full Spinal Stretch

Lift and hold the tail at an angle that creates a natural continuation of the spine, so the vertebral joints are not compressed above or to the side. If you could look down from above, your horse's head and spine would ideally be in a straight line to get the most benefit from this exercise. Your horse may bend her neck to see what you're up to – verbally ask her to straighten it as you begin to lean your weight backward and create the stretch. Send her a mental image of her straightened body pulling away from you. Your horse will most likely straighten her head and neck the first or second time that you do this, enjoying its full benefit. A helper can gently encourage her to do so.

It's very important that both of your hands hold on to bone, not just hair. Plant your feet firmly, one widely spaced in front of the other. Keep your back straight, your shoulders relaxed, and your arms straight and aligned with your horse's entire spine. Slowly lean your weight back into your back hip as you bend that knee, holding firmly onto the tail bone. Lean your whole body weight to create as large a stretch as you can. Your horse should respond by leaning her weight forward, away from you, creating the stretch with you (Photo 21.5). Photo 9.6 on page 59 shows Katydid stretching her entire spine from the last tail vertebra through her poll and even down through her jaw, in response to Pamela's backward pull; her head and spine and Pamela's arms form a straight unbroken line.

Hold for five to ten seconds. Release very, very slowly so that there is no compression. You may hear little cracking sounds – the release of fluid in the joints, which is of no concern.

This stretch imparts a great feeling of wholeness, sending energy from one end of the body to the other and out to the limbs and organs through the meridians and nerves. Horses obviously appreciate and enjoy it. For these reasons, it is one good way to end a session, even a short one. Stroking would still follow as your last technique.

22 *Index of Specific Problems*

These techniques are **not** intended to replace proper diagnosis and appropriate treatment by a veterinarian and/or farrier.

Arthritis

Shiatsu techniques must be applied very carefully to arthritic conditions. A "less is more" principle is to be used.

As most arthritis involves degeneration of the joint surfaces, manipulation could further aggravate the process. When there is inflammation, direct pressure and manipulation could worsen the condition, bring too much blood to the area and increase the swelling. In all cases, work the entire body (as described in SHIATSU TREATMENT: A Shiatsu Massage: Diagnosis and Treatment, p. 89) to balance the energy, and *avoid* the distressed areas. If swelling is absent or subsides, the area may be *gently* moved by rotation, stretching and jiggling.

The principle to remember when treating arthritic conditions (which include navicular) is that you need to drain energy out from the area; you do not bring energy to it, as through pressure stimulation or a holding palm. Gentle rotations, stretches and jiggles will help to move and release the energy. You may also use specific point pressure on the terminal meridian points of the feet (Photos 18.3a–b): this will draw the energy down and out. Use a steady holding pressure with your thumb, either until you feel the point quite activated, or for as long as feels comfortable to you and your horse. You might pay particular attention to the terminal points of the Heart Constrictor and Kidney Meridians, located at the posterior centers of the feet in the hollow between the bulbs of heel. The Kidney Meridian, by the way, supports the health of the bones.

Applying shiatsu generally and regularly, particularly along the Bladder Meridian, should theoretically stimulate the endocrine system and the immunological response to help slow the degenerative process and, perhaps, halt bony overgrowth. Acupuncture can be effective in this way. Herbal and nutritional supplements may be helpful.

Colic – early or mild indications, or while waiting for your veterinarian

Use pressure technique on the ears, as described in SHIATSU TREATMENT: The Head, p. 106. Firmly press the tips of the ears. You can do this repeatedly, and while you are walking your horse.

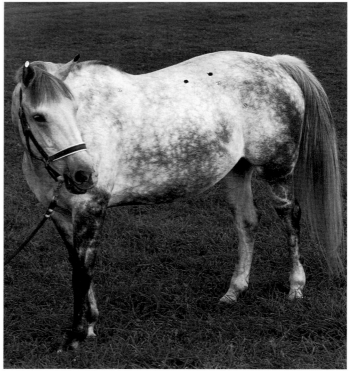

22.1 Some beneficial tsubo points for colic.

Use specific, firm thumb pressure on the other two points indicated in Photo 22.1. These are located on the upper path of the Bladder Meridian, in the groove of the longissimus dorsi muscle. The first is at the junction of the thoracic and lumbar vertebrae. The second is centered above the tuber coxae. Repeat pressure as needed. These are the association points for the Stomach and Large Intestine Meridians. You may also work along these meridians.

Hind-leg stretches, first forward, then rearward, will relax the abdominal muscles, which may have a positive effect on the intestinal tract.

Eyes — runny with tears or mucus

Massage the tear-duct and use the techniques for the eyes that are described in SHIATSU TREATMENT: The Head, pp. 104–105.

Founder and Laminitis

Lifting a leg will place too much stress on the standing one. Use thumb pressure on the meridian lines in the legs. Give particular attention to the Heart Constrictor and Triple Heater Meridians. If excessive heat is present, work from the foot upward; otherwise, work downward towards the ground. With your thumb, seek to locate points where energy feels depleted: hold these for several seconds, or wait until you feel some response (a sensation of energy beneath your pressure).

Work for a few minutes on each leg, alternating back and forth.

You may do three half-hour sessions each day.

Headaches

Many people suspect that their horse has a headache. It's in the way the horse looks around the eyes, or in her jaw, or in the way she carries her head. The discomfort may be due to allergies, a misaligned neck vertebra, fatigue, jaw tension, or even anxiety.

Give gentle neck shiatsu. Gradually increase your degree of pressure each time you move down the neck along the three lines of meridians. Work each side four or five times, alternating back and forth. Work the poll area, holding points a few seconds longer.

Work the ears. Rotate each in both directions, holding between your thumb or index finger in front and your other fingers behind, as you support the head with your other hand. Then press the point of the ear between your thumb and fingers as you lift the ear slowly out from its socket, in four directions. You may work one ear at a time or both simultaneously.

Apply fingertip or thumb pressure to the forehead, moving upward, then outward. Slowly work the eye sockets. Work the mouth and jaw, first wetting your hand if the mouth is dry inside. To relieve jaw tension, repeat the technique of pulling and stretching the cheek muscles (with thumb inside and fingers outside of the mouth).

Rotate the skull within the joint of the first cervical vertebra. With a supporting hand over the poll, use your other hand under the chin to do slow and small head rotations or side to side movements. With one hand still on the poll and the other hand on the nose, press the nose slowly downward toward the chest, hold for five to ten seconds, and slowly release before removing your hands.

If you have time, work the Bladder Meridian and stretch the tail. Then, leave your horse alone to relax.

Inflammation

This is an over-accumulation of energy and fluids as the body rushes to repair damage. Often it is painful to the touch.

With a very relaxed arm, wrist and hand, the fingers of your hand touching together, and your arm moving loosely in the shoulder socket as though it's hanging from it, make large back and forth or circular sweeping motions, passing your hand a few inches in front of the inflamed site. It's all right if your elbow is bent, but your arm must be relaxed. This motion sweeps away the disturbed energy and allows cool, fresh, healing energy to flow in. You may need to do this repetitive

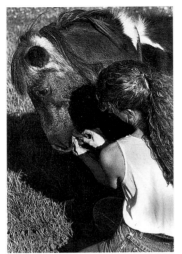

22.2a *We're working to overcome this pony's 25 year old habit of constantly nipping and licking. Pamela's right, "supporting" hand gently and firmly holds his lower lip down and away from his teeth. Her "moving" thumb, of her left hand, presses at the base of the gum where it curves into the lip. Pressure is applied and released rhythmically all long the gum line. Stardust is fully absorbed in the sensations being created.*

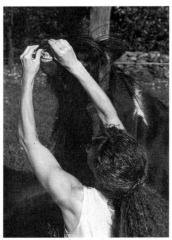

22.2b *Both hands can work simultaneously, if your horse is as complying as our pony. The thumb and index finger press the lip while gently pulling it out; they then release, move on and repeat.*

movement for approximately one hour, but it need not be all in one session. Until you are used to the motion, your arm will probably tire, so do as much as you can in a series of sessions until you feel the swelling has disappeared.

Lameness — undiagnosed

(1) Watch your horse move, from behind, beside and in front of her, and move with her (see TECHNIQUES: Evaluating Problems, p. 37).
(2) Work the Bladder Meridian of the back, looking for sore spots. Press to test around the point of hip, the hip joint, the stifle joint, and the point on the buttock where the hamstring attaches.
(3) Work the Bladder and Gall Bladder Meridians in the hind legs.
(4) Work the front and back lines of the shoulders, and the elbows.
(5) Sensitively work each leg, front and/or hind, beginning with foot rotations. Work *upward*, testing each joint for reactiveness.
(6) Stretch the tail to each side, looking for tightness or resistance. This will show you if one side of the back is stiffer.
(7) Stretch the neck to both sides.
(8) Check for tension at the poll. This may indicate head pain and/or emotional tension, both of which can affect the entire body.

"Mouthiness" — nipping, biting, licking, orally fixated

Pressing on the tsubos of the gums and stretching the cheek muscles work to allay annoying mouthy habits, such as licking, nipping and biting. Horses with these habits can be very quickly distracted out of them by these techniques, which also stimulate, relax and, in time, by repeated application, can reduce or eliminate the habits. (I was very impressed by a stallion's model temperament, including an atypical lack of mouthiness. Then his owner showed me how she plays with his lips and gums — unknowingly, by instinct, she was using shiatsu.)

Gums

Use the techniques for the lower and upper gums on p. 102 of TREATMENT: The Head. In addition, gently but firmly hold the lip away from the teeth with one hand as the thumb of the other hand presses at the base of the gum, where it curves into the lip (Photo 22.2a). Pressure is applied and released rhythmically along both the upper and lower surfaces, moving from one side of the mouth to the other. Release and watch as your horse mentally and physically absorbs this unusual kind of attention.

Lips

Hold the inner and outer surface of the lip between your thumb and index finger. Press with gentle firmness and release, working rhythmically from one side to the other as you did over the gums. You can gently pull and massage the lip as you press (Photo 22.2b).

Cheeks

Stretch the cheeks as in the technique on p. 102. Then gently "pinch" the cheek between your thumb and fingers, about level with the mouth, and pull it slightly outward. Repeat in two more positions, moving upward towards the nasal bone (Photo 22.2c).

Match your speed, rhythm and degree of pressure to your horse's energy. Our pony, in the photos, is a bit erratic and neurotic, and so the above techniques were done with quick, firm pressure. This distracted as well as relieved his mouthy urgings. For a calmer horse you would slow your movements and perhaps use lighter pressure.

Navicular

Work the foreleg meridians, particularly the Heart Constrictor, with specific thumb pressure. If there is heat in the foot, or an excess accumulation of energy, work from the foot upward. Pay particular attention to pressing the points on the foot (see illustrations of the tsubos of the feet, p. 119 – the points are the same on the fore and hind). The HC terminal point of the foot lies in the hollow between the bulbs of heel. Knock on the hooves, with knuckles or the end of a crop, to encourage circulation.

Also work the entire body to balance the horse's energy and allow her to regain a sense of wholeness. The longer a horse spends in the navicular/founder stance, the stiffer she will become – first in the shoulders and back, then through the hindquarters. Working the Bladder Meridian will rebalance the energy and relieve stiffness and soreness

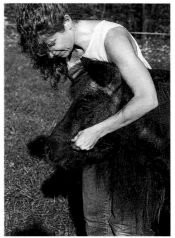

22.2c Gently "pinch" the cheek between your thumb and fingers and pull it slightly outward.

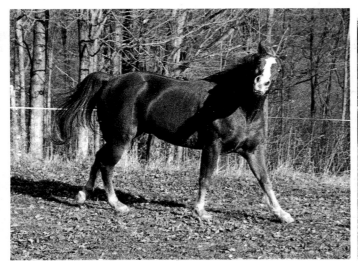

22.3a Red wears egg bar shoes and wedge pads, but a year or two of the "navicular pose" made his entire body stiff, painful and constricted. He moved entirely on his forehand, crooked, with short steps and an inverted back.

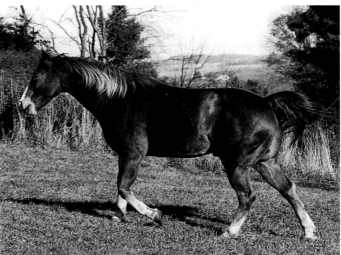

22.3b After three fifteen minute shiatsu sessions, Red's profile in motion has markedly changed: his movement is straight and lengthened, his spine is coiled (notice that his back is raised), he's less on the forehand and using his hindquarters.

accumulated along the back. Working the hindquarters will renew flexibility and take the horse's attention (and weight) off of the forehand. Stretching the tail and spine will release blocked energy and impart a sense of wholeness. (See Photos 22.3a—b, showing Red before and after treatment.)

Maintain her energy in balance and her sense of wholeness. Work the meridians of the forelegs and feet when pain seems present.

As much as is possible, you want the horse to carry herself properly – using the ring of muscles through the back and the hindquarters, and staying flexible and relaxed through the neck and shoulder. Correct riding and basic dressage techniques to develop flexibility and correct development of the muscles will help.

Corrective shoeing will often relieve pain and reduce concussion to the area. The feet should be kept well trimmed at the proper angles. Herbal and nutritional supplements may help. Acupuncture may help to halt or slow down the degenerative process and to relieve pain.

Shock, Trauma, and After Surgery

Keep your hands on your horse as much as possible, touching, stroking, and reassuring with your voice as well as touch.

Make sure your horse hears your own deep, even breathing. This will encourage the same from your horse, and ensure that *you* remember to breathe and center your attention.

Use the stroking technique. Use whatever other techniques seem feasible and applicable in the situation. You want to remember to:
○ rebalance the energy;
○ restore circulation;
○ dissipate heat and inflammation.

Use pressure along the meridians, and other moving energy techniques, such as percussion. Keep your pressure even and firm – if you're too gentle, your horse may not feel you in a shock situation. You may want to use a deep or quick distracting pressure.

The point GV 26 is used for shock and loss of consciousness. It is located on the midline between the base of the nostrils. Use firm, deep pressure.

The homeopathic remedy **arnica** is administered for shock, trauma, and surgery.

"Tying-up"

Speak reassuringly to your horse as you work.

Work the Bladder, Gall Bladder and Liver Meridians, using deep pressure and prolonged holding of points. You might use elbow pressure in this case, particularly over the hindquarters and buttocks.

Stretch the tail side to side, and rotate each vertebra of it by manipulating the space between the bones (gently), bending them side to side and up and down. Lift and arc each vertebral joint, in succession from the dock. Stretch the tail: lean back, release slightly, lean back a bit more, release slightly again, then lean back and hold the stretch for ten to fifteen seconds, or more if the horse seems comfortable and is participating by leaning away from you, straightened, in the opposite direction.

Rework the meridians, especially from the hip through the hock.

Use gentle, cupped-hand percussion on the buttocks and hamstring muscles.

Jiggle the neck, by holding over the crest and gently rocking it to and fro – the head should softly swing in the opposing direction. Do "standing jiggles" of the front legs (without lifting them).

Use the stroking technique.

Now attempt to walk your horse. Repeat all of the techniques if necessary.

Lastword

Perspectives

The horses stand at the gate. "Where have you been?" ask their eyes and ears.

"I've been writing."

"What's that?"

"It's my art of arranging words – the sounds you hear me think to express the ramblings of my mind – so many other humans may know them."

"Primitive!" they say with a twist of lips and narrowed eyes.

"Humans aren't horses," I remind. "We're a relatively new species, still trying to figure things out."

The thought "too much figuring" takes form within, as I catch my mare's mischievous grin and glint of eye.

Marion Kaselle, 1992

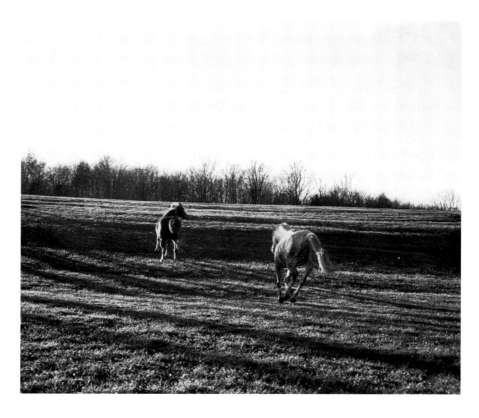

Appendix A

Notes on the Twelve Major Meridians

Each meridian is a complex system of associations, both physical and emotional. The book *Traditional Acupuncture: The Law of the Five Elements* explores the personalities of the meridians. Pamela, reluctant to assign the same emotional associations from humans to horses, has compiled the list of emotional attributes in the following "Symptoms Index of Meridian Correspondences" from her direct observations and careful considerations.

Some associated qualities result from the physical location of the meridian in the body. For example, the Bladder Meridian, located along the back and the back of the hindquarters and the hind legs, is associated with impetus, or the lack of impetus, which in extreme cases becomes fear. Some emotional correspondences stem from physical symptoms associated with a meridian. A horse with sinus problems, congestion and difficult breathing – all physical problems of the paired Lung and Large Intestine Meridians – will have trouble interacting with other horses, since a sense of smell also serves their social interactions. It follows that a horse reacting to the irritants of a new environment could become distressed and withdrawn. The associations of the emotional symptoms are logically based.

YinYang theory

Each of the twelve major meridians is defined as either Yin or Yang and coupled accordingly with another meridian that is supportive and complementary in function. The meridians on the outside of the legs are Yang, while those on the inside are Yin. The sun's energy of heat and brightness is said to be Yang, and the earth's energy is said to be Yin. Because the sun touches the back and the sides of the body, the meridians located in these areas are Yang. And because the energy from the earth comes up to the body's underside, the meridians there are Yin. Three major meridians in the horse somewhat contradict these given rules: the Large Intestine, a Yang meridian, runs on the inside of the lower leg; the Stomach Meridian, also Yang, runs on the underside of the chest and abdomen; the Heart Meridian, which is Yin, runs just to the outer side of the horse's lower leg and ends on the outer foot.

The Ki energy in the Yang meridians, on the outside of the legs, moves downward (from the sun to the earth); in Yin meridians, on the inside of the legs, Ki moves upward (from the earth towards the sun). The YinYang flow of Ki is charted on the human with the arms raised to the sky, and this same model is used with four-legged animals. In other words, to know the YinYang flows by the principles given (Yang moves from sun to earth, and Yin from earth to sky), picture your horse with his front hooves raised to the sky.

Traditional Oriental medicine seeks to move energy in the natural direction of its flow, according to the laws of YinYang. But some forms of practice move the energy from the interior of the body outward to the extremities. There are exceptions, of course, within rules of practice. One example is dammed energy: when the foot is inflamed, you want to move the pooled energy back up the leg to restore circulation and a balanced energy flow.

The study of YinYang is extensive, and it is difficult to make generalizations. Even within a single cell there is Yin and Yang, inseparable, but separately identifiable. The tree you see above the ground is obvious Yang and its unseen roots are Yin; but root vegetables are considered Yang, and leafy vegetables Yin. What is important to remember is that Yin and Yang are always mutually supportive and inseparable, as a tree with its roots. The Ki flowing through each Yin meridian and each Yang meridian must have YinYang balance for health.

1994 Postscript

Through my own practice of Chi Kung, Chi Healing and acupressure, I now have answers and insights into many of my own unanswered questions. I've gained these by actually feeling the energy flows within the meridians, vessels and organs, within myself and within my patients. My treatments now are entirely orchestrated by the energy of my patient – not by my will, nor analytical decisions, nor intuition, but by my contact with the self-healing directive of the energy of that individual. My arms and hands and at times my entire body are moved by the individual's energy to move, remove and put in energy. Working in this way throws out all "rules" save those inherent in the life force. Some insights from this way of working are:

○ Chi (Ki) flows in whichever direction is needed for healing. Often I move energy alternately in both directions to release a blockage.

○ A healthy bodymind continuously inhales fresh, high-frequency energy through the acupoints and body pores and releases excess or disturbed energy in order to maintain balance, health, and to increase vitality. Giving treatment, I sometimes remove energy by first moving fresh energy in, directing its flow, then moving out the disturbed and excess.

○ Pressure on points and along meridians directs the flow of energy; it can also open points for energy to enter and exit. Press and release of the fingers on a point informs and allows the energy to adjust as needed; holding a point gives warmth and support, not healing energy, unless you've developed the ability to simultaneously bring it into yourself and send it out.

○ Traditional Chinese Medicine names sets of points through which to significantly increase and release energy. In humans, those to increase energy occur at the wrists, elbows, ankles and knees; in horses they circle the knees, elbows, hocks and stifles. The Baihui point of the Governing Vessel, GV20, located at the poll joint, also increases energy. Points to readily release energy are, in humans, on the fingers and toes, and in horses on the coronary band of the hooves and around the base of the fetlocks. I also often use the following points both to add and remove energy: GV1 and CV1, above and below the anus; GV2 – on the underside of the tail about two inches from the tip; GV26, at the base of the nostrils, and CV24, at the base of the lower gum (you can press from outside of the mouth).

The **Five Elements Theory** sits at the core of Traditional Oriental Medicine. We originally considered it beyond the scope of this book, and would refer you to innumerable books on it. It is valid and extremely valuable as a diagnostic guide. I hope that those of you wanting to pursue this course will seek its wisdom.

Symptoms Index of Meridian Correspondences

MERIDIAN	FUNCTION	PHYSICAL Associations	EMOTIONAL Associations
LARGE INTESTINE YANG front feet	Reception and elimination	Infections, fever Digestive disorders, colic Breathing passage constriction, nasal congestion	Anti-social behavior, difficulty adapting to new environment
LUNG YIN front feet		Respiratory problems Sinus problems Allergies Infections	Grief
STOMACH YANG hind feet	Digestion, transformation and distribution	Colic, digestive disorders Overeating or poor appetite Flatulence; Bad breath Sinus congestion	Nippiness, anxiety, excessive curiosity
SPLEEN YIN hind feet		Digestive problems, colic, diarrhoea Loss of appetite, overeating Blood and circulation disorders; excessive bleeding Muscle soreness Reproductive problems	
SMALL INTESTINE YANG front feet	Circulation of blood	Colic Inflammation	Tendency to over-exert, over-do Emotional, over-reactive Sad
HEART YIN front feet		Fever Fatigue Circulatory problems	Unhappy about relationships (horse or human)

MERIDIAN	FUNCTION	PHYSICAL Associations	EMOTIONAL Associations
Bladder YANG hind feet		Nervousness General fatigue Hind-leg soreness and stiffness Headaches Neck pain Back pain	Reluctance to move forward Fear of going into new environment Headstrong Aftermath reaction to stress
	Storage and elimination of essence and fluids	Fluid retention Bladder disorders Clamped tail	
KIDNEY YIN hind feet		Fatigue, weakness Lumbar pain Fluid retention Bladder disorders Reproductive problems Hormonal imbalance	Fear Depression
TRIPLE HEATER YANG front feet		Shoulder joint problems Hormonal imbalance Hoof (forelegs) problems	
	Circulation and protection	Founder Fever	Emotional, over-reactive Sad
HEART CONSTRICTOR YIN front feet		Circulatory problems Hoof (forelegs) problems Founder Fever	Unhappy about relationships (horse or human)
GALL BLADDER YANG hind feet		Joint, tendon and ligament problems Hip lameness Hind-leg lameness General muscle soreness	
	Storage and regulation	Headaches Neck tension	Mental inflexibility, stubbornness Anger
LIVER YIN hind feet		Muscle strain and inflammation Hind-leg stiffness Circulatory problems Eye problems	

Superficial Pathways of the Twelve Major Meridians and Two Vessels

The accompanying diagrams and their descriptions are based on the meridian charts by Meredith Snader, VMD, current Executive Director of the International Veterinary Acupuncture Society.

The **Large Intestine Meridian** begins just above the coronary band at the medial center of the forefoot. It goes up the medial center of the pastern, to the medial posterior of the cannon and splint bones to the base of the knee. It then moves across the front of the knee to the lateral side of the leg, follows a muscle groove from the lower anterior edge of the radius to an indentation at the lower end of the humerus (level with the elbow). It follows the anterior of the humerus and the groove of the brachiocephalicus muscle – just above the pectoral muscle, then just above the jugular groove to the end of the groove. It then crosses the lower and upper jaws to terminate outside the lower portion of the nostril.

A.1 Large Intestine Meridian (continuous line), and Lung Meridian (dashed line).

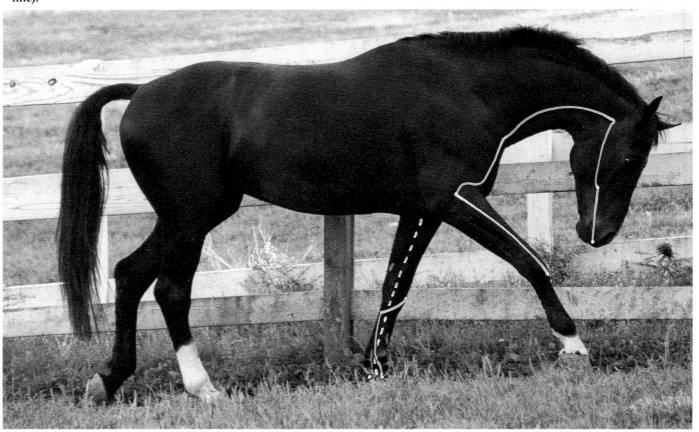

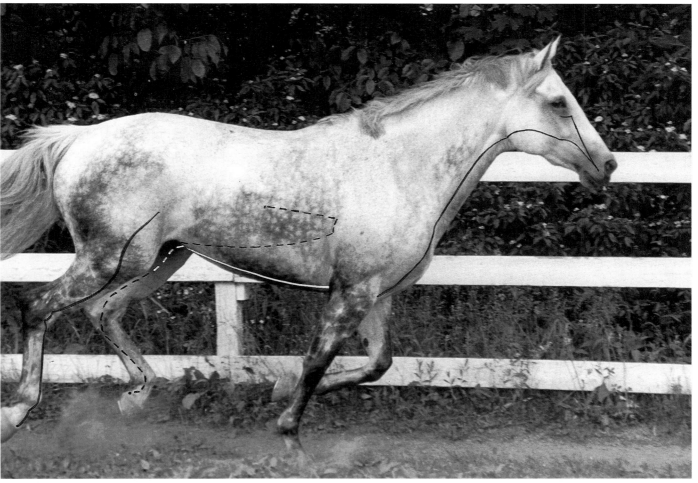

A.2 Stomach Meridian (continuous line) and Spleen Meridian (dashed line).

The **Lung Meridian** begins in the lungs, emerges at the most anterior point of the third rib (just above the anterior-medial foreleg), then down to the costal cartilage, and down the medial center of the leg, ending on the inner bulb of heel.

The **Stomach Meridian** runs from the indentation below the midline of the eye, through the upper jaw to the gums of the mouth, back through the lower jaw, to and down the lateral edge of the sternocephalicus muscle of the neck – just below the jugular groove, then down the chest along the inside groove of the major pectoral muscle. It travels along the belly about a handswidth from the ventral midline, and passes through the leg to an indentation at the flank. It moves straight down the muscle groove, through the anterior of the stifle joint to the depression just below it on the tibia bone, then down the anterior of the tibia and upper hock. At the middle hock, it moves to the anterior center of the leg, and so down the lower leg to terminate just lateral to the anterior center of the coronary band of the hind foot.

The **Spleen Meridian** begins on the inner bulb of heel of the hind foot, goes up the medial center of the pastern and metatarsal bones to and through the middle of the hock, then up the posterior edge of the tibia and stifle. It crosses over to and up the side of the abdomen, to the posterior edge of the fourth rib – about level with the point of shoulder, then back across the lateral center of the ribs to the posterior of the fourteenth rib.

The **Small Intestine Meridian** begins just above the lateral center of the coronary band of the forefoot, goes up through the lateral center of the pastern, to the posterior of the bones of the lower and upper leg, around the point of elbow, to a depression at the posterior of the lower humerus, then straight up to the posterior edge of the scapula. It now zig-zags forward and slightly down to the center of the spine of the scapula (the protruding vertically centered ridge), up to the scapula's dorsal anterior edge, and down to above the first thoracic vertebra. It then goes up the neck to the joint between the second and third cervical vertebrae, over the lower border of the atlas to the lateral base of the skull, and around the lateral side of the ear to the end point in the depression in front of it.

A.3 Small Intestine Meridian (continuous line) and Heart Meridian (dashed line).

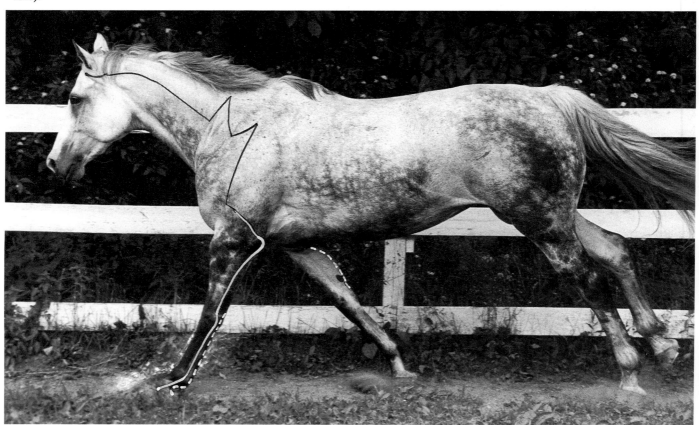

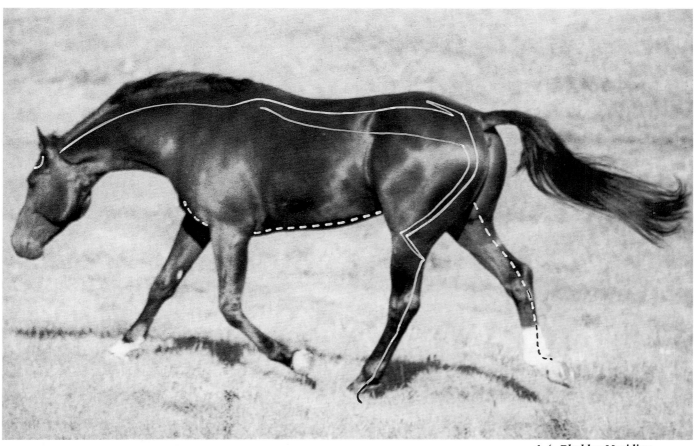

A.4 Bladder Meridian (continuous line) and Kidney Meridian (dashed line).

The **Heart Meridian** begins at the heart and emerges deep behind the elbow in the horse's equivalent of an "armpit". It goes to just medial of the posterior center of the upper leg. At the top of the knee joint it passes to just lateral of the posterior center, continues so to behind the fetlock and down the pastern, and ends on the outer bulb of heel.

The **Bladder Meridian** is described in detail on pp. 89–99.

The **Kidney Meridian** probably begins at the apex of the frog on the bottom of the hind foot. It has a point at the posterior center of the foot in the hollow between the bulbs of heel. It goes then to the medial posterior edge of the pastern, over the fetlock to the medial posterior edge of the metatarsal bones, through the center of the hock, up just posterior to the tibia, and up the inner leg to the abdomen. It travels across the abdomen and up the lower chest two fingerwidths from the ventral midline, to a point between the sternum and the base of the first rib.

The **Triple Heater Meridian** begins just lateral of the anterior center of the coronary band of the forefoot. It goes up the lateral anterior of the pastern and the base of the cannon, passing to the lateral center and through the center of the knee, up the center of the radius, over the base of the humerus to its posterior side, forward to the posterior of the shoulder joint, to about two-thirds up the anterior edge of the scapula, up the neck passing over the first four cervical vertebrae, to behind the ears and the base of the skull, then around the medial side of the ear, and finally to a point in the depression above the eye.

The **Heart Constrictor Meridian** begins in the lining of the heart, emerges just above the inside of the elbow, goes to the center of the medial side of the leg, passes over the chestnut, then down the posterior edge of the radius. It continues down the medial posterior edge of the leg bones, passing in front of the accessory carpal bone of the knee. From the pastern it moves to a point at the posterior center of the foot in the hollow between the bulbs of heel. It probably goes from here to the apex of the frog.

A.5 Triple Heater Meridian (continuous line) and Heart Constrictor Meridian (dashed line).

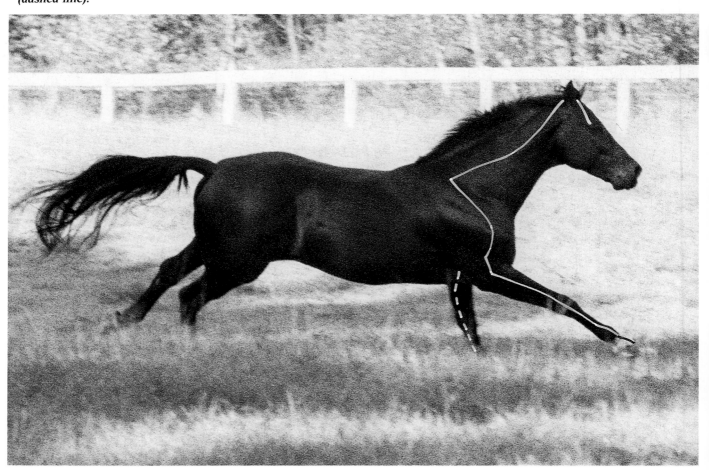

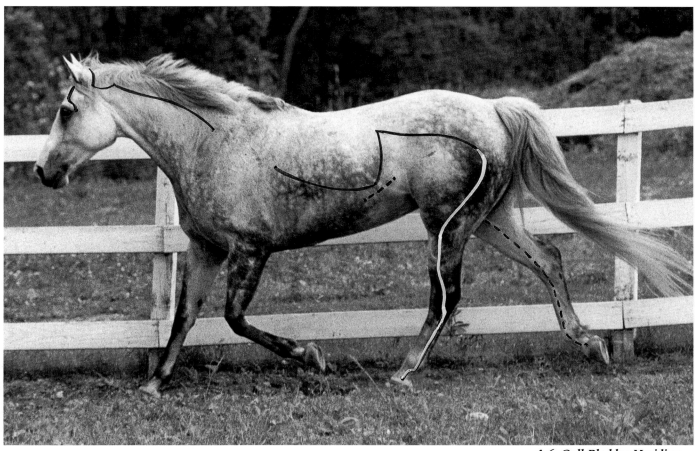

A.6 Gall Bladder Meridian (continuous line) and Liver Meridian (dashed line).

The **Gall Bladder Meridian** begins at the outer corner of the eye, goes up around the medial side of the ear and the back of it to the lateral base of the skull, then over the atlas and second cervical vertebra, and down the upper part of the neck (closely below the Bladder Meridian) to the dorsal anterior of the scapula. It now runs internally and reappears posterior to the shoulder muscles and the sixth rib. It goes to near the base of the fifteenth rib, to posterior of the middle of the last rib, runs below the tuber coxae over to the hip joint, then to the major trochanter of the femur, down the posterior side of the femur, to and down the center of the tibia, through the center of the hock, down the posterior edge of the metatarsal bones, and forward down the center of the pastern to terminate just above the lateral center of the coronary band.

The **Liver Meridian** begins on the hind foot above the medial center of the coronary band, goes up the medial anterior of the pastern, cannon and hock, then up the center of the tibia and stifle joint and the inner leg. It then moves internally, comes out at the base of the last rib, and goes finally to the base of the fourteenth rib.

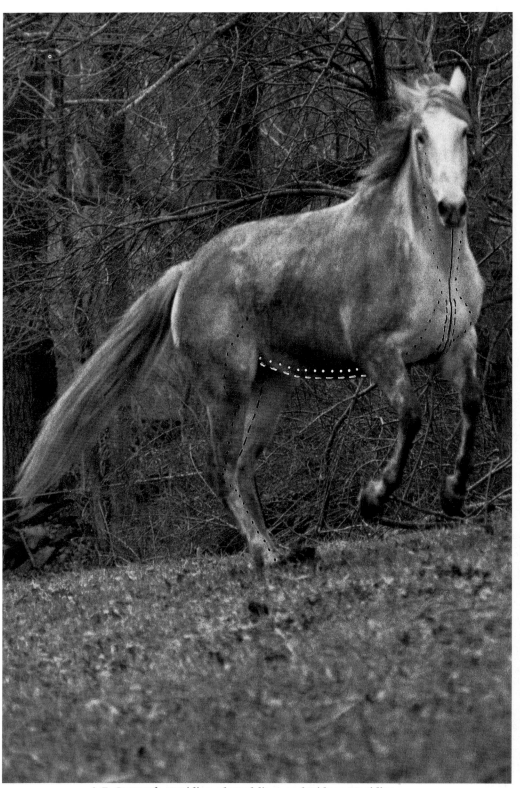

**A.7 Stomach Meridian (dotted line) and Kidney Meridian
(dashed line) and Conception Vessel (continuous line).**

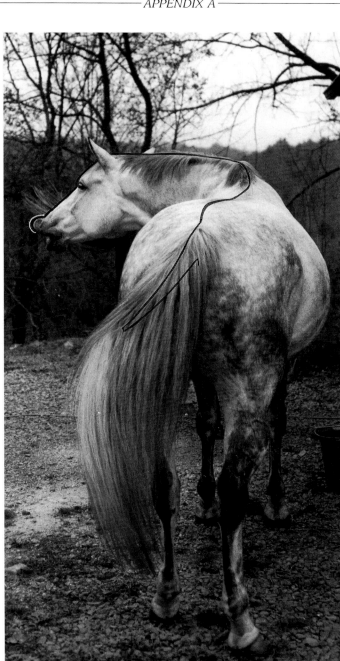

A.8 Governing Vessel.

The **Governing Vessel** begins in the hollow below the base of the tail, traces the bottom of the tail bones to the tip of the last vertebra, then the dorsal midline of the body to the center of the upper gum of the mouth.

The **Conception Vessel** begins below the anus and follows the ventral midline of the body to the center of the lower gum, from where it connects to the Governing Vessel.

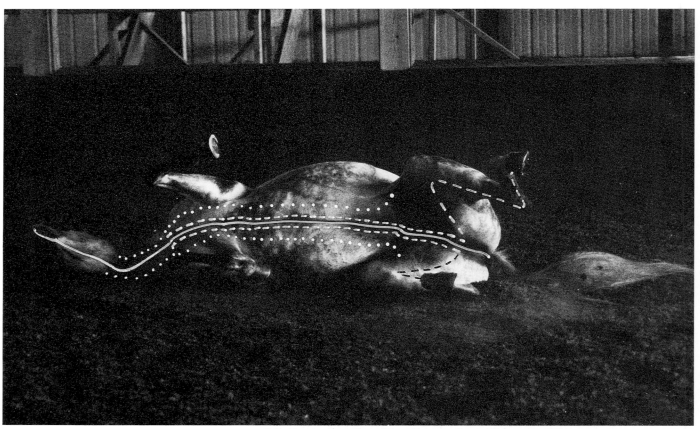

A.9 Conception Vessel (continuous line), Kidney Meridian (dashed line) and Stomach Meridian (dotted line).

Appendix B
Holistic Medicine in Veterinary Practice
with
Allen M. Schoen, DVM, MS

Allen M. Schoen has a DVM from Cornell University, a MS in neurophysiology and behavior from the University of Illinois, and is certified in veterinary acupuncture and chiropractic care. He is the past-president of the International Veterinary Acupuncture Society, and author of the latest textbook on the subject, *Veterinary Acupuncture*. He is on staff of the Animal Medical Center in New York City, the largest animal hospital in the world, where in 1982 he established a department of veterinary acupuncture. While maintaining an acupuncture and alternative-therapy referral practice, half small animal and half equine, much of his time is devoted to teaching and research. He is one of the primary instructors of the International Veterinary Acupuncture Society's post-graduate certification course, and he lectures throughout the world to veterinary organizations and conferences as well as to horse and dog clubs. He is the founder of VITA (Veterinary Institute for Therapeutic Alternatives), an institute for research and instruction.

Holistic medicine seeks balance, a balance encompassing all aspects of the patient. When we speak of balance, we are mindful of the Chinese concept of YinYang, the inseparable polarities that, when in balance, ceaselessly flow together, transforming one into the other. We apply this concept to many aspects of health in animals.

The first goal of holistic health care is prevention. We look at the entire animal, within his entire environment, and apply the principles of balance. We look to the horse's nutritional and health needs. We consider the balance of his physical body, maintaining structural alignment, feet trimmed to the proper angles for the individual's conformation, the rider's balance, and a properly fitting saddle. The horse's mental balance must be maintained as well, by consideration of his environment, caretakers and training demands.

The physical balance of the rider and between the rider and the horse must be considered. If the rider is out of balance, not straight and centered, has a subluxated hip, or a back problem, and rides crooked, the horse will eventually show signs of corresponding soreness and misalignment. This may cause the horse to favor one leg and develop a lower leg problem. The leg will demand treatment, but the primary problem of the rider's imbalance will remain as a continuous aggravation. If the horse is misaligned or otherwise unbalanced, from another cause, his rider may develop misalignments of the back or hip, become unbalanced through attempting to maintain balance with the horse. Both, in their natural drive to find balance, will compensate and compound the originating problem.

Training must be balanced between the physical and mental capacity of the animal and the demands made upon him. You must consider his conformation and suitability for the tasks given, as well as his physical and mental development and condition of the moment. If a horse says "No", you must discover the **why** behind it, evaluate rather than push.

The environmental needs of horses will affect their mental balance, and therefore the balance of the whole. They have a need for adequate space, light, ventilation, company, and a view. A small, dark, dull "jail cell" will depress a horse and impact on his personality, his tractability and his health.

When you consider balancing the needs of the entire animal, you are practicing preventive and holistic medicine. Many equine veterinarians recommend a medical preventive-health program. In addition, when a problem does arise – an emergency, a traumatic injury, or just something unforeseen – you call your regular veterinarian for a diagnosis and evaluation of the situation. The first consideration is the animal and what form of treatment will best fulfil his very individual needs of that moment. We here speak of the balance between Eastern and Western medicine. Not one of them has all of the answers, or nothing else would exist. We need to recall the YinYang flow and see that Eastern and Western medicine complement each other, work together, flow one into the other. The art of being a good physician or veterinarian is not in just making the diagnosis, but in knowing which therapy is most appropriate for that condition in that individual. It may be surgery or antibiotics or other drugs, or it may be acupuncture or chiropractic or shiatsu or homeopathy or nutrition, or a combination of any of these.

Alternative therapies often address problems and circumstances lying outside the realm of conventional medicine. Shiatsu, herbal remedies and nutrition have preventive as well as curative benefits. These therapies along with acupuncture and homeopathy can enhance healing as an adjunct to conventional treatment. At times, as in an emergency, homeopathy and shiatsu may be beneficial as you await the arrival of your veterinarian. Then there are situations where conventional medicine does not produce results, or does not have a reasonable approach to the problem, or cannot make a diagnosis because the problem does not show up on the routine physical/lameness examination or on x-rays.

Veterinarians certified in alternative therapies offer a different perspective. The conventional veterinarian, like the general practitioner, makes the evaluation and diagnosis. When the situation is judged to be outside the confines of conventional treatment, as with certain musculoskeletal problems, the alternative treatment may be appropriate. The horse is then examined and diagnosed according to the techniques of traditional Chinese acupuncture, and/or chiropractic examination. Homeopathic and/or herbal remedies and/or nutritional supplements may be prescribed as the prime treatment or as an adjunct. Often shiatsu and massage techniques are prescribed as follow-up and preventative measures.

Dr Schoen: "My concern with lay people reading a book and learning shiatsu is that they might tend to use that instead of going the extra mile when it's needed and having acupuncture or chiropractic done, or they might call in a massage therapist when the animal actually needs more than that. And that's the question of judgement. A book like this is an invaluable contribution to the equine literature and self-help for animal owners. However, there's a balance, and one needs to be cautious that if you're concerned at all that you're not sure what's going on, you don't continue massaging your horse when something else such as acupuncture, chiropractic or conventional medicine may be more appropriate and accelerate the healing of your horse. The main concern for all of us is the animal healing the best way he or she can."

Acupuncture

Acupuncture is the stimulation of specific points on the body to achieve a homeostatic or therapeutic effect. Based on traditional Chinese medical theory, homeostasis is the proper energetic balance of Yin and Yang. Acupuncture is used to diagnose and treat any imbalance of Chi (Ki).

Acupuncture is now known to affect all major physiological systems. It works primarily through the central nervous system, affecting the musculo-skeletal, hormonal and cardiovascular systems. It does more than relieve pain. Acupuncture increases circulation; causes a release of many neurotransmitters and neurohormones, some of which are endorphins, commonly known as the body's "natural pain-killer"; relieves muscle spasms; stimulates nerves; stimulates the body's defense systems; as well as numerous other beneficial effects.

Acupuncture has been used successfully for nearly four thousand years on animals as well as humans. It is still the treatment of choice for one quarter of the world's population for many problems. In the Western world, it is used primarily when medications are not working or are contra-indicated due to possible side-effects, or when surgery is not feasible. In China, it is often used as the primary treatment prior to conventional medicines and surgery.

For horses, acupuncture is most commonly used to treat:
○ musculo-skeletal problems (back problems, navicular disease, laminitis, tendonitis, and numerous other lamenesses);
○ nervous disorders – traumatic nerve injury;
○ analgesia – for surgery;
○ respiratory problems – heaves, "bleeders".
Treatments may last from ten seconds to thirty minutes, depending upon the condition treated and the method employed. There are many

ways to stimulate acupuncture points, including the insertion of needles, electro-acupuncture, aquapuncture (injection of a solution into the point), moxibustion (heating the point), and laser acupuncture. Patients are often treated one to three times a week for four to six weeks. A positive response is often noticed within the first four to six treatments, sometimes earlier, depending on the condition treated. Because acupuncture balances the body's own system of healing and no chemicals are administered, complications rarely, if ever, develop.

Chiropractic Care

Chiropractic focuses on the health and proper functioning of the spinal column. The spinal column of the horse is a complex structure made up of bones, ligaments, muscles and nerves. It provides the framework of support, muscle attachment, protection of the central nervous system, and protection of internal organs.

A **subluxation** is the chiropractic term for a misaligned vertebra that is "stuck", or unable to move correctly. Subluxations cause stiffness, resistance and lessened ability. They also disrupt nerve transmissions, the flow of information between the brain and the cells of the body, especially where nerves exit between two vertebrae. Problems may arise in nerves that supply other cells such as those of the skin, glands and blood vessels. Obstructed nerve transmission to the muscles will impair normal co-ordinated movement, which will cause at the least a slight lessening of performance, at worst a damaging mis-step. Nerve pressure also causes pain. Compensation to avoid pain increases the stress and the problems.

An **adjustment** is the veterinary chiropractor's attempted correction of a misalignment. It is a short, rapid thrust directly on the vertebra, very specifically directed to replace it in a normal position. A controlled force is used. Simply because horses are large does not mean that abnormally large forces are needed to adjust them. The joints of the spine are moveable, and if the correct angle is used, the adjustment is relatively easy and of low force. Veterinary chiropractors may also manipulate the joints of the legs, as well as the jaw. Although it is a diverse field, and there are many different types of techniques, most will use only their hands to adjust the vertebrae of horses. The adjustment releases the "stuck" vertebra and restores alignment, thus eliminating nerve pressure. The body can then repair tissues and restore function.

The muscles and ligaments of the horse must be able to maintain the correct spinal alignment. Healing takes time. Several adjustments may be needed until the body accepts and maintains the correction. Most horses will show significant improvement in one to four adjustments. However, chronic spinal problems take longer to respond. Horses who are basically sound and engaged in work suited to their conformation will respond quickly and maintain spinal alignment for a longer period of time.

Homeopathy

Homeopathy is a medical science discovered in the early 1800s by Samuel Hahnemann, a German physician and pharmacist. It is a formal system of drug therapy based on principles often diametrically opposed to those in orthodox medicine.

The drugs of homeopathy, called **remedies**, are derived from plants, animals, minerals, bacteria, viruses, disease products, chemicals, hormones, and more. They include many substances that, in their natural state, are poisonous, and some that are biologically inert until they are prepared in the homeopathic method.

Homeopathy is based on the "Law of Similars" that "like cures like". Remedies are prescribed according to their **provings** of producing in healthy persons symptoms similar to those of the patient. It is a truly holistic medicine. Treatment is based on a whole picture of the patient. The physical, emotional and mental characteristics are equally considered to see the total pattern of symptoms. This pattern is matched with the remedy that produces the same or similar complex of symptoms. The symptoms of the disease itself are often the least important when selecting a remedy.

Another principle of homeopathy lies within its method of preparing the remedies. The method is called **potentization**, and it creates the **microdose**. Through a process of serial dilution, and each step being accompanied by vigorous shaking, called **succussion**, the original substance is increasingly diluted, *and potentized*. A decimal dilution is indicated by x or D ($6x = 1/1,000,000 = 10^6$), a centesimal dilution by c or cH ($6c = 10^{12}$); $1M = 10^{2000}$. Once the dilution of $24x$ (which $= 12c$) is reached, no molecules of the original substance will remain, yet with each dilution and succussion, the potency of the remedy is *increased*. The rule of homeopathic remedies is: the higher the dilution, the greater the potency. This is totally opposite to orthodox pharmacology, where greater potency comes from higher molecular concentrations. The process of potentization apparently liberates and intensifies the energy latent in the original substance. The active agent of the potentized remedies is its subtle energy signature.

Homeopathy, as acupuncture and shiatsu, cures through activating the natural healing process within the individual on the subtle energy level. This is why they say, "Treat the patient, not the disease." Underlying the homeopathic precepts is the principle of the **vital force**, the energetic life force synonymous with Chi of Chinese medicine, prana or kundalini of Indian yoga, and the orgone of Reichian theory. Disease is seen as a disturbance of the vital force, originating on the subtle energy level, resulting in symptoms on the molecular plane – dis-ease of the physical, emotional and mental body. The potentized remedies work by the energy form or frequency of the substance stimulating and rebalancing the vital force energy of the patient, who will then self-heal.

Unlike orthodox drug therapy which is often designed to suppress symptoms, homeopathy views symptoms as expressions of a curative process, the body's attempt to regain balance. This process is the body's way to rid itself of toxins. Therefore, the remedies promote the symptoms in order to complete the process. A "healing crisis" is sometimes created in the initial stages of treatment, during which the condition is aggravated and symptoms intensified, after which the illness resolves itself. When symptoms disappear, or there is marked improvement, treatment is ceased.

There is a list of remedies proved useful, often invaluable, in first-aid situations. It is a good idea for horse owners who use alternative therapies to keep a homeopathic first-aid kit in their barn and with them when they travel with their horses. The remedies apply equally to the same symptoms in humans and animals, and in many acute first-aid situations the same high potencies can be used. A suggested list is given on p. 178.

The remedies most commonly come as sugar tablets, and are dissolved under the tongue. It is very important to avoid contamination – their tube or bottle should be kept well sealed, away from excessive heat, and, when dispensed, the pills should not contact anything other than their container's cap. An easy way to administer to horses and avoid contamination is to dissolve the tablets in one or two teaspoons of *distilled* water and squirt under the tongue with a syringe.

It is advisable in cases other than first aid to consult a veterinarian trained in homeopathy. Homeopathic prescription is an art as well as a science. The experience and insight of the physician are as important as knowledgeable training. Firstly, the correct remedy to match the patient's symptoms must be found, or there will be no response. Then the right potency and the frequency of dosage must be determined. The American Holistic Veterinary Medical Association (or in Great Britain, the British Association of Homeopathic Veterinary Surgeons) will supply the names of veterinarians trained in homeopathy. The addresses are given at the end of this appendix.

References

There are numerous introductory books to be found. There are two books available specifically for horses:

G. MacLeod, *The Treatment of Horses by Homeopathy*, The C.W. Daniel Co., Saffron Walden, England, 1984.

G. Emich, *Naturopathy for Horses*, J.A. Allen and Co. Ltd, London, England, 1994.

Suppliers of remedies

United States

Many health-food stores are now carrying homeopathic remedies. The following members of the American Association of Homeopathic Pharmacists are among those who supply mail-order catalogs:

Boericke & Tafel, Inc.
1011 Arch Street
Philadelphia, PA 19107
215-922-2967

Luyties Pharmacal Company
4200 Laclede Avenue
St Louis, MO 63108
800-325-8080

Boiron-Borneman, Inc.
6 Campus Boulevard
Building A
Newtown Square, PA 19073
800-258-8823

Dolisos America Inc.
3014 Rigel Street
Las Vegas, NV 89102
800-365-4767

California only

Boiron-Borneman, Inc
98C W. Cochran Street
Simi Valley, CA 93065
800-258-8823

Canada

D.L. Thompson Homeopathic
  Supplies
844 Yonge Street
Toronto 5, Ontario
M4W 2H1

Great Britain

Ainsworth's Homeopathic
  Pharmacy
38 New Cavendish Street
London W1M 7LH

A. Nelson & Co. Ltd.
73 Duke Street
London W1M 6BY

Horses' Homeopathic First-aid Kit

*THESE REMEDIES ARE NOT MEANT TO REPLACE VETERINARY DIAGNOSIS AND TREATMENT, BUT TO **ENHANCE HEALING**.*

Arnica 30c: shock, trauma, wounds, bruises, injury of any sort, muscle spasm, muscle inflammation – 2x, 2–3 hours apart; (HUMANS: for same – 3x, $\frac{1}{2}$ hour apart, then 1–3x/day if symptoms persist);
ointment: topically on swellings.

Hypericum 30c: nerve injuries – 1x/day for 1 week;
(HUMANS: crushed toes and fingers – same as Arnica).

Aconitum napellus 30c: laminitis – every 30 minutes for 6 doses;
fear – $\frac{1}{2}$ hour before riding.

Apis 6x, 6c or 30c: bug bites – 2x/day with symptoms;
wind galls – 4x, 1 hour apart.

Arsenicum alb. 30c: allergic dermatitis – 1x/day for up to 10 days;
1M: dry dermatitis – 1x/day for 1–2 weeks.

Belladonna 6c: fever – every hour until fever goes down.

Calendula ointment: skin healing, for a large area or chronic non-healing wound.

Ledum 6c: punctures – 4x, 2 hours apart;
mosquito bites – 1x when bitten.

Nux vomica 6c: colic – every 2 hours for 4 doses;
1M: laminitis – every 2 hours for 4 doses.

Rhus tox. 30c: inflammatory arthritis – night and morning for 4 days;
1M: osteoarthritis – 1x/day for 1 week.

Rhus venenata 30c: photosensitivity – night and morning for 4 days.

Ruta grav. 6c: sprains – 3x/day for 3 days.

Thuja 30c: vaccinations (to counter adverse reactions) – 1x/day for 1 week, beginning day before vaccinated.

Dosage: 4–6 tablets or pillules of high potencies (30x–200x, 30c–200c, 1M)
5–10 tablets or pillules of low potencies (6x–24x, 6c–12c)

Pour from cap or sterile vial to directly under the tongue, or dissolve in 1–2 teaspoons of *distilled* water and squirt under the tongue. Do not allow pills to contact any other surface, including your hands. Never return unused pills to their container if they've contacted anything other than their own dispenser cap. Reclose container immediately. No food or water should be given for twenty minutes before or after administration of remedy.

Cease treatment when there is marked improvement.

Herbal Remedies

Although herbal medicine lies historically at the very roots of modern drug therapy, they diverge with the reductionism of Western medicine. Western pharmacology isolates the one most active chemical within the healing plant, then replaces it with a synthetic version. Herbal medicine looks holistically at the healing power of the individual plant. There are many substances within the plant. Herbalists believe that the therapeutic elements are contained in more than just the primary acting chemical constituent, and that they cannot be separated from the whole. The whole is further considered to have an individualized energetic profile vital to the healing complex.

Herbal remedies do not directly attack disease, as Western drug therapy is designed to do. Rather, the herbs direct the patient's own healing potential to cure the disease at its origins.

Chinese herbs are formulas of *combinations* of herbs, minerals and animal products. The herbs or other natural substances combined within a formula complement and build on one primary herb or substance, and prevent any side-effects. They can have profound effects without the side-effects of synthesized drugs.

American herbs are usually used individually, not in combination. There are many available, such as yucca, and aloe vera, that have particular benefits. Many of these are now marketed specifically for horses. One of these is yucca, which has been known to help arthritis and navicular. Many "old home remedies" really work, and in situations that conventional medicine doesn't always have good answers for.

The question with herbal remedies for horses is whether the preparation contains pharmacologically active doses. Herbs must be given in sufficient quantity for the active ingredients to be effective. You must read labels very carefully for the percentage and weight of the primary herb.

Reference recommendation
Juliette de Bairacli Levy, *Herbal Handbook For Farm and Stable*, Rodale Press, Emmamus, PA, and Faber and Faber, London, 1976.

Nutritional Supplements

We're increasingly finding that our animal feeds are missing certain vitamins or nutrients, due to deficiencies in the soil, or shipping, or age, or some other cause. Often our animals need additional vitamin and mineral supplementation for deficiencies in the local pasture or feed supply, or for their level of work.

The veterinarian may determine by blood analysis, history and physical examination, by Western diagnosis and Chinese diagnosis, the existence of certain deficiencies and need for specified supplementation.

Alternative Veterinarian Referrals

You may locate a veterinarian trained and certified in the respective alternative therapies by writing to the societies listed below, and enclosing a self-addressed, stamped envelope.

United States

International Veterinary Acupuncture Society
RD #1
Chester Springs
PA 19425

American Veterinary Chiropractic Association
PO Box 249
Port Byron
IL 61275
Tel: 309-523-3995

American Holistic Veterinary Medical Association
2214 Old Emmorton Road
Bel Air
MD 21015

Great Britain

Association of British Veterinary Acupuncture
85 London Road
Guildford
Surrey
Tel: 0483 573199

Institute of Complementary Medicine
Unit 4
Tavern Quay
London
SE 16
Tel: 071 237 5165

British Chiropractic Association
29 Whitley Street
Reading
RG2 0EG
Tel: 0734 757557

The McTimoney School
The Institute of Pure Chiropractic
14 Park End Street
Oxford
OX1 1HH
Tel: 0865 246687

British Association of Homoeopathic Veterinary Surgeons
c/o Christopher Day
Chinham House
Stanford-in-the-Vale
nr Faringdon
Oxon
SN7 8NQ
Tel: 0367 710324

References and Suggested Reading

'Animals', *Parabola*, Vol. VII, No. 2, New York, May 1983.

BERGER, JOHN, *About Looking*, Pantheon Books, New York, 1980.

BOONE, J. ALLEN, *Kinship With All Life*, Harper & Row, New York, 1954.

CHOPRA, MD, DEEPAK, *The New Physics of Healing* (audio cassette), Sounds True Recordings, Boulder, CO, 1990.

CHOPRA, MD, DEEPAK, *Quantum Healing Workshop* (audio cassette), Sound Horizons Audio Video Inc., New York, 1990.

CONNELLY, DIANNE M., *Traditional Acupuncture: The Law of the Five Elements*, The Center for Traditional Acupuncture, Columbia, MD, 1979.

DAVIDSON, JOHN, *Subtle Energy*, The C.W. Daniel Company Ltd, Saffron Walden, England, 1987.

ELLENBERGER, W., H. BAUM AND H. DITTRICH, *Animal Anatomy*, ed. by Lewis S. Brown, Dover Publications Inc., New York, 1956.

GALLWEY, W. TIMOTHY, *The Inner Game of Tennis*, Random House, New York, 1974. [Author's note: this book is about "being here now".]

GERBER, MD, RICHARD, *Vibrational Medicine*, Bear & Company, Sante Fe, 1988.

HEARNE, VICKI, *Adam's Task: Calling Animals by Name*, Alfred A. Knopf, New York, 1986.

MACLEOD, C, MRCVS, DVSM, *The Treatment of Horses by Homoeopathy*, The C.W. Daniel Co. Ltd, Saffron Walden, England, 1984.

MASUNAGA, SHIZUTO, WITH WATARU OHASHI, *Zen Shiatsu*, Japan Publications Inc., Tokyo and New York, 1977.

MOSKOWITZ, MD, RICHARD, *Homeopathic Reasoning*, San Francisco, paper presented at the Symposium "Homeopathy: The Renaissance of Cure", March 29, 1980.

OHASHI, WATARU, *Do-It-Yourself Shiatsu*, E.P. Dutton, New York, 1976.

SWAMI VISHNUDEVANANDA, *The Complete Illustrated Book of Yoga*, Bell Publishing Company, New York, 1960.

WESTERMAYER, DR MED. VET. ERWIN, *The Treatment of Horses by Acupuncture*, translated by Dr Ac. D. Lawson-Wood & J. Lawson-Wood, The C.W. Daniel Co. Ltd, Saffron Walden, England, 1979.

YANG JWING-MING, DR, *The Root of Chinese Chi Kung*, YMAA Publication Center, Jamaica Plains, MA, 1989.

ZUKAV, GARY, *The Dancing Wu Li Masters: An Overview of the New Physics*, William Morrow and Co., Inc., New York, 1979.

Index

Page numbers in *italics* refer to illustrations.